Empowering Parenting Techniques for Down Syndrome Kids

Bessie .M Berry

Funny helpful tips:

Cultivate a sense of wonder; it keeps the spirit young and vibrant.

Respect each other's space; individual time is essential for personal growth.

Empowering Parenting Techniques for Down Syndrome Kids : Effective Strategies for Parenting Children with Down Syndrome to Foster Growth and Independence

<u>Life advices:</u>

Seek feedback regularly; it's a tool for growth and self-improvement.

Maintain clear documentation; it's crucial for audits and compliance.

Introduction

This is a comprehensive resource for parents who have a child with Down syndrome or who have recently received a prenatal or birth diagnosis. The guide covers various stages of the journey, starting from the early stages of diagnosis through adulthood.

The Basics section provides an understanding of what Down syndrome is, the types of diagnoses (prenatal and birth), and the initial emotions and challenges that parents may experience upon receiving the diagnosis.

The Journey section is divided into different age groups, focusing on specific developmental milestones and challenges faced by children with Down syndrome and their families. It covers the following stages:

1. Newborn to Six Months: This stage provides guidance on early infant care, addressing health concerns, and establishing a strong bond with the baby.
2. Six Months Through Two Years: This section focuses on developmental milestones, early interventions, and therapies that can support the child's growth and progress.

3. Ages Three Through Five: Here, the guide discusses preschool and early education options, socialization, and preparing for primary school.
4. Primary and Middle School: The guide addresses education, inclusion in mainstream classrooms, and social interactions in the primary and middle school years.
5. Teenage Years: This stage covers the unique challenges and opportunities that arise during adolescence, including education, self-advocacy, and transitioning to adulthood.
6. Life for Adults with Down Syndrome: This section explores the various paths that adults with Down syndrome may take, including vocational opportunities, independent living, and community engagement.

The "You Are Not Alone" section emphasizes the importance of support and community for families with children with Down syndrome. It provides information on Down syndrome support groups, organizations, and research initiatives that can connect parents with valuable resources and a worldwide network of friends who understand their journey.

Overall, this book aims to empower parents with information, guidance, and support to ensure they can provide their child with the best opportunities and experiences throughout their life with Down syndrome.

Contents

Chapter One
What *Is* Down Syndrome?

Whether you are looking for scientific specifics or general information, resources abound to gain a better understanding of Down syndrome. Your first instinct will probably be to go to the Internet. Although you can find a lot of important information there, be careful about accepting all of it as true. Diverse opinions and thoughts, not all well informed, spread across your computer screen.

Instead, focus upon resources that provide current, complete information. Look for materials that show the celebrations and the struggles. Like anything in life, Down syndrome involves a wide range of experiences.

Facts about Down Syndrome:

- Down syndrome is a common genetic condition involving the twenty-first chromosome.
- There is no known cause of Ds.
- Ds can impact every cell in a person's body or just some of them.
- It is more often diagnosed in babies of older mothers. However, Ds happens with parents of all ages, races, religions, and socioeconomic backgrounds.
- According to the National Institutes of Health in 2012, about 1 in every 700 babies is born with Ds.
- In the United States, about 5,000 babies are born each year with Ds.

- Every person with Down syndrome has areas of strengths and challenges.
- People with Ds may also experience:
    - Heart defects
    - Hearing loss
    - Hypothyroidism
    - Alzheimer's
- There is a wide range of abilities, behaviors, and development in people with Ds.
- Adults with Down syndrome can have jobs, drive cars, live independently, and get married.

NOTE FROM THE AUTHOR

When I first Googled the words "Down syndrome," I found *lots* of information. I found bulleted lists of all the medical conditions that could possibly come with Down syndrome. I found amazing stories about accomplishments by people with Down syndrome. I found stories of fear about Down syndrome. It was really difficult to picture our son in any of those realities. Then I found parent blogs—ones that were honest, real, and raw. These families shared about the celebrations and the challenges in daily life. Those blogs gave a much fuller picture of our potential future. Search and research as much as you'd like (you know you will!), but also take it all with a grain of salt and remember that no one can predict anyone's future—including that of your family.

—Jen

Hearing "the Words"

Down syndrome. Most parents can recall the moment when they were told their child might have Down syndrome. Your background knowledge and life experience play a large role in how you receive and process the news, but regardless of how and when the diagnosis was delivered, there are common thoughts you share with every other parent of a Ds child. As you begin to research and watch your child grow, you will discover what Down syndrome means for your child and family.

Here are some thoughts from parents of children with Down syndrome about when they first heard the news:

"I had zero knowledge of T21, as she was a birth diagnosis and all my thoughts were old and dusty."

"I assumed I was doomed to spending the rest of my life navigating an unintelligent person through the basics of life."

"I thought it was hereditary. I thought there were mild and severe cases. I thought they weren't able to do anything for themselves."

"We are doomed! This is the *worst* thing ever! Life is over."

"I thought I was being punished by God. I would be stuck with kids forever and me and my husband would never enjoy vacations or retirement."

"Having grown up with a close friend who has Ds, I knew of the potential! I wasn't afraid."

"I have always been accepting of all people with special needs. In high school I was a counselor for summer camp for two weeks for people with all sorts of special needs. But even with the experiences I have had . . . it was still very scary."

"I know nothing about this and now it is our life."

"I wondered what on earth we just did to our older daughter's life."

"People with disabilities made me uncomfortable. I grew up *very* sheltered in a small community with very few disabled people. Whenever I was around someone, I was very uncomfortable because I knew nothing about them and how I was supposed to treat them."

"I thought I caused it. Maybe it was that margarita I had when I didn't know I was pregnant yet . . ."

"My first fear was that she would never know how much I love her, how much her family loves her."

"I thought of my aunt who was sweet and loved art and fashion."

"I was never taught to be accepting of all people as my mom was always very judgmental of other people. I am ashamed to say she passed that on to me to a degree. I was devastated. I knew *nothing* about Down syndrome."

"My very first thought about Ds, when I found out our son had it, was people are going to be mean to him. I cried for months over this thought."

Advice to New Parents

Jenna Strauss has mosaic Down syndrome, and she loves to talk about her life experiences. She and her boyfriend of several years recently went their separate ways, but she has a new cat to keep her company, as well as her music like Def Leppard. Advice she would give new parents: "Be optimistic and just be with them every step of their way, especially when they start struggling! Get involved with the school and see if there are any clubs that they can join. Those of us with Ds can easily be affected emotionally. If someone starts bullying them, be there for them. Don't let them see your fear and mostly you'll feel inspired when they start doing things on their own!"

What Are the Types of Down Syndrome?

There are three different forms of Down syndrome, each with its own characteristics and manifestations of the twenty-first chromosome.

1. *Trisomy 21*—At conception, each cell has three copies of the twenty-first chromosome. This is the most common form of Down syndrome.
2. *Translocation Down syndrome*—Very early in pregnancy, part of the chromosome attaches to another chromosome. People with translocation Ds have two copies of the twenty-first chromosome and another part of a twenty-first

chromosome attached to another. This is a genetic condition that can be hereditary.

3. *Mosaic Down syndrome*—Mosaic Down syndrome (mDs) occurs when not all cells have an extra copy of the twenty-first chromosome. For those with mDs, there can be a wide range of cells affected.

The only way to know which form of Ds your child has is through bloodwork and the karyotype report that will analyze the individual chromosomes from your child's DNA.

OUR EXPERIENCE: Translocation Down Syndrome

We learned our daughter has translocation Down syndrome when we received her karyotype results. She had a birth diagnosis, so at that point we were still trying to regain our footing and understand what all of this meant. We decided to take a few months to consider whether we wanted to know if one of us was a translocation carrier. Ultimately, we chose to find out because of the possible impact on future pregnancies. Balanced translocation carriers have higher rates of miscarriage as well as an elevated chance of having a child with Down syndrome. I'm very much a "need to know" kind of person, so it just felt right to know if one of us is a carrier. When our daughter was six months old, we found out that I am a balanced translocation carrier. Having this type of Down syndrome does not change anything about what we might expect with an extra chromosome, but it does make for interesting conversations with genetic counselors! I think it is a bit special to know that my sweet girl and I share a translocated chromosome!

—MELISSA STOLTZ

Does It Matter?

You may be wondering if it really matters what type of Down syndrome your child has. In fact, it does. There are few distinctions, other than future genetic implications, between trisomy 21 and translocation trisomy 21. Mosaic Down syndrome (mDs), however, can present in different ways and depends a lot on which cells carry the extra chromosome. Cases of mDs can often go undiagnosed for years. Translocation trisomy 21 can be hereditary, so further genetic testing may be pursued by families for the purpose of future family planning.

Karyotype

A karyotype of your child's chromosomes will confirm a Down syndrome diagnosis. In pregnancy, samples of cells or fluid are taken prenatally during a chorionic villus sampling (CVS) or amniocentesis. After birth, the doctor will take a blood sample from your baby and send it to a nearby laboratory. Once at the lab, the DNA is analyzed and a photograph is produced of the chromosomes. Typically each person has forty-six chromosomes. People with Down syndrome have an additional twenty-first chromosome (or partial chromosome) for a total of forty-seven. The results of your child's karyotype will be shared through a report from your child's doctor or genetic counselor and will include details about your child's DNA and recommended steps for you to consider.

OUR EXPERIENCE: A Mosaic Diagnosis

I was twenty-three when Lucas was born, a perfectly healthy boy at eight pounds eleven ounces and twenty-one and a half inches long. Things took an unexpected turn at seven months when he began eating stage 3 baby foods. Before, he ate well and put on weight, but things changed, and Lucas was diagnosed with "failure to thrive." We were all stumped. Lucas began early intervention and worked on oral motor skills. He improved some but not enough to put our minds at ease. Multiple times his doctor asked if we were interested in genetic testing and multiple times we stubbornly declined. Finally, just before Lucas's eighteen-month well-child visit, yet another sick visit, and following surgery for a set of tubes in his ears, we agreed to genetic testing. We waited for three weeks and received a call from the doctor to come in for a visit without Lucas. Our hearts dropped. We sensed that our lives were about to take a different direction and nothing could have prepared us for what the doctor had to say. "Lucas has something called mosaic Down syndrome." My husband and I were lost in the words "Down syndrome." Since then, Lucas has proven to us, and many others, that Down syndrome, mosaic or not, was never something that would keep him down. No one in our lives has ever taught us as much as Lucas has about love, hard work, and compassion.

—BRANDY SNOW

International Mosaic Down Syndrome Association (IMDSA)

IMDSA is designed to support any family or individual whose life has been touched by mosaic Down syndrome. The organization pursues research opportunities and increases awareness in the medical, educational, and public communities throughout the world. There are many ways that it accomplishes this mission, including:

- Research and Retreat Weekend, held annually in the United States
- Annual photo campaign that highlights individuals with mosaic Down syndrome
- Toll-free hotline available for individuals to connect with IMDSA
- Multiple social media and Internet-based forums and environments
- Research scholarships for researchers doing genetic studies
- Genetic toolkit for researchers and medical professionals
- Professional booklet with information about mDs

The group also acts as a resource for local Down syndrome associations to help ensure that the organizations are best equipped to serve those affected by mosaic Down syndrome in their communities.

OUR EXPERIENCE: How Does Mosaic Down Syndrome Impact My Daily Life?

At seven, speech communication [with our son] is our biggest struggle, and that is something that we work with each and every day. While it does sometimes cause frustrations (for all of us), Jared's created his own strategies to be understood through pictures, sign language, and now even spelling! The other big impact for us is that since his "Ds-ness" doesn't show in his typical facial appearance, it's not easily apparent to others why he doesn't communicate well or why he may act a little differently than the other kids. This leaves me with an awkwardness of if, when, and how to explain our unique situation. If I had known when we first got the mDs diagnosis at eight months, just how "normal" most of our days are living with a seven-year-old who has mosaic Down syndrome, maybe I wouldn't have been so scared.

—JENNIFER SMOLKA

Welcome to the Community!

Or, as the award-winning author and mother of a child with Down syndrome, Emily Perl Kingsley, said, "Welcome to Holland" in her poem, "Welcome to Holland," Kingsley used the metaphor of taking a fabulous trip to an unexpected destination as a descriptor of her experience and emotions connected with discovering the new journey brought on by having a child with Down syndrome. (*www.our-kids.org/Archives/Holland.html*). (Dear Parents, if you haven't yet read/heard this short poem: Do. Even if you don't love it, someone in your circle will.)

Every parent's needs and access to a community of support are unique. Parents looking for parent-to-parent support can start in a variety of places. Here are several:

1. Down Syndrome Diagnosis Network (an online and local support network connection for families with children under three): *www.dsdiagnosisnetwork.org*

2. BabyCenter Down Syndrome Boards: *http://community.babycenter.com/groups/a315/down_syndrome*
3. International Down Syndrome Coalition (a support network connection for all ages): *http://theidsc.org*

Finding a Local Group

You can also connect with your local Down Syndrome Association (DSA). Local groups are discussed more at length in Chapters 4 and 10. However, for a start you can find via the National Down Syndrome Society a list of local affiliates here: *www.ndss.org/Resources/Local-Support*. The Global Down Syndrome Foundation has a listing of local resources as well: *www.globaldownsyndrome.org/about-down-syndrome/resources/local-organizations*. Sometimes your doctor or hospital will have information about local organizations that can be helpful as well. Still need help? Contact DSDN for help finding families near you.

Get the Support That's Right for You

What support looks like varies from person to person. Your priority is to look for resources that offer up-to-date information and parent/family connections. Do not feel compelled to join or share your experiences if it makes you uncomfortable; ease in as is right for your family. Some parents jump right in to advocacy and campaign immediately with local and national groups. Others need time to focus exclusively on their child and family and adjust to their future and their emotions. They often benefit from the support of one or two new friends to help them through the process. Both of these methods are correct.

"Special Children to Special Parents" and Other Misnomers

Parents sometimes feel too overwhelmed to talk to other parents; they don't understand why they got "chosen" for this gig. Before your child was born, maybe you looked at parents of children with special needs and thought, I could never do that! Or, that mother is so patient, or, that father is so strong. And now . . . that's you!

How did you get this job when you're *so* underqualified? Impatient? And anti-angelic? Well, now you know the secret. That magic wand you thought parents of special needs get—they don't. It's true: No parent really knows how this whole thing works. Talk to other parents and realize they are just like you. We're all winging it. None of us are "special parents" with special qualifications that got us this job. Parents, like every parent in the history of mankind, have done nothing more special than creating a new life. (Okay, that *is* pretty special.) People will now say to you how special you are to have a child with Down syndrome. You may smile and nod, like the millions of parents who are with you in the club, knowing that you're just as qualified, or unqualified, as the next person.

Don't let your previous image of a "special needs parent" keep you from connecting with other parents, who are, in fact, flawed humans, too. "Just meeting real, live, other parents can be emotionally and practically reassuring that you are not alone and that you can do this, whatever the 'this' seems to be," says Brian Long, Connor's dad.

Information Overload

Often new parents jump on the research wagon out of a furtive desire for *the answer*—the definitive information that will make everything fall into place. Remember that part of support is supporting yourself. Give yourself time to love, to breathe, to enjoy, to celebrate, to recover, to share, and to just live. Jisun Lee, the mom of a toddler nicknamed LP, says to new parents, “Anyone who knows me can tell you that I’m something of an obsessive researcher. Yet, on this, I have to go the other way and say that I think what has given my family an advantage is not so much the research, but the times I’m willing to fly without it. Sometimes, a parent needs to listen to that little voice inside and jump without knowing that there are double-blind scientific studies to back them up, you know? Sometimes, a parent needs to do what they know is *right*, even if research reveals that he or she is in the minority.”

NOTE FROM THE AUTHOR

When my son was born, there wasn’t *really* an Internet, but there were books. I read those books. For two weeks I took in as much information as I could absorb. Then my sweet son did what the books said he *shouldn’t* be able to do—he rolled over. He rolled over from front to back. His doctor didn’t believe me, but so what? He did this and it was real. So I threw all the books out the window. No book could or would ever be able to tell me what Marcus can or can’t do. Period. As an author of this book, I suggest you do the same. If you find yourself reaching “information overload,” if the information is stressing you and not helping you, throw this book through the window and enjoy your family, first and foremost.

—*Mardra*

Obligations, Terminology, and Important Dates

So often at community events, family members and educators of children and adults with Down syndrome share that one of the benefits of having a child with Ds in your life is the opportunity to connect with other great families with such a strong sense of community. Now that you're *in the club*, you should be aware of some of the obligations, terms, and important dates.

Obligations

The only true obligation is to your child and your family. Within the community there are various networks of support and advocacy, but—this may surprise you—there remain widely different opinions and ideas about advocacy, education, and awareness, and the best way to get to the end game: the person with Ds living a long and fulfilled life.

Just as many have preconceived ideas about people with Down syndrome, so people also bring to the table previously held notions about *the parents and families* of those with Down syndrome. Diversity reigns! So, to be clear, your first and only true obligation is to the well-being of your child with Down syndrome. What we, as the authors of this book, and what your local and national organizations hope to achieve, is to provide you with the tools, awareness, and support necessary to get you and your family to that goal. No two families have ever chosen, or will ever choose, the exact same path.

Terminology

The first way you can become an advocate for people with Ds is simple: You can start using People First Language. As explained on this website, *www.disabilityisnatural.com/explore/people-first-language*, People First Language describes the conscious use of language to both avoid and prevent the dehumanization of people with disabilities. In the case of people with Down syndrome, there are two primary "rules" to consider.

1. A person has Down syndrome—a person is not Downs; there are no "Downs babies" or even "Downs parents." For example, my son, Marcus, has Down syndrome. He is not a Ds person or a Down's child.
2. Someone with Down syndrome does not "suffer from" Ds and should not be described in this way.

Language evolves, and consequently people, even professionals, may not consider or be aware of usages that are offensive. Educate yourself and your family, then gently work to educate others and encourage them to use People First Language.

Already you may be finding your own word choices changing. You may discover your growing sensitivity to what was once a medical term, then slang, and is now regarded as hate speech: the "R-Word." As we said, language evolves, and even the federal government is starting to make changes. For example, in 2013 the Social Security Administration announced they were replacing the term "mental retardation" with "intellectual disability" in their Listing of Impairments used to evaluate claims involving mental disorders. Other parts of the federal government are taking similar steps.

English versus English

In 1974, the U.S. National Institutes of Health declared that the condition would be called Down syndrome (instead of Down's syndrome), declaring, "the author (John Langdon Down) neither had nor owned the disorder." In the UK, the correct language is still Down's syndrome. As Hayley Goleniowska points out in her advocacy blog *DownsSideUp.com*, "Neither is wrong and respect is paramount . . . Now, let's work together to ensure a great future for our kids . . . Let's work together to support each other, whether our kids have Down syndrome or Down's syndrome. What is important is our message and the drive to communicate that."

Calls to change the way people refer to others with intellectual disabilities are supported by the national Down syndrome groups as well as the Special Olympics and R-Word.org, which hosts the "Spread the Word to End the Word Campaign." Changing the words people use requires changing their attitudes, and remains an ongoing challenge. One dad, Rob Snow, decided to try to help other parents with the honest and funny book *What I Should Have Said*. Snow, who is also a standup comedian and motivational speaker whose life opened up when his son with Down syndrome was born, recognized the times he *wished* he said something alongside all the ways he's learned to help others understand the power of words. He suggests helping people to see individuals and their unique gifts, and choosing humanity instead of throwaway words. He educates people across the country in order to facilitate changes in their language and outlook.

Important Dates/Events

You will soon find out, thanks to social media, that there are times within the Ds community that are more active. Two important times both nationally and internationally are March and October. Although there are other activities sprinkled throughout the year, this is when we share with the world all about Ds.

World Down Syndrome Day (WDSD)

This is a global awareness day that has been officially observed by the United Nations since 2012. It is celebrated on March 21 each year. (3-21. Get it?) Down Syndrome International hosts the WDSD website "to create a single global voice for advocating for the rights, inclusion and well-being of people with Down syndrome on 21 March." Each year international Down syndrome organizations and advocates gather with self-advocates, educators, government officials, and medical professionals at a one-day conference held in the UN. The conference is shown via live webcast and the previous years are available for viewing as well on the WDSD website.

MY STORY: DEVON ALDERMAN

In 2015, Devon Alderman, a teenager with Down syndrome, was one of the several self-advocate speakers. Here is the transcript of her speech before the audience at the United Nations:

"In primary school I learned letters and learned to read. I also started my love for marine life. In middle school I had lots of fun in classes, sports, and plays. I had fun with friends, too. Now I am in high school. I'm a cheerleader, a soccer player, and an 'A' student. My favorite classes are video production and marine biology. I will graduate in June. I love learning and also I love sharing.

"After I graduate I'm going to college. I hope to work in the field of marine biology. I want to live in an apartment and maybe someday [with] a husband. I deserve to be up here talking to all you guys. Thank you for making me feel very included today. Being included is being awesome. Thank you." The complete presentation including her parents, Sean and Susan Alderman, is available via The Road We've Shared website.

***

National Down Syndrome Society Buddy Walk on Washington

This event, hosted by NDSS, is held each spring and is aimed toward supporting people with Down syndrome through legislative advocacy. Self-advocates and parents converge on Washington DC to discuss issues and speak to members of Congress.

National Down Syndrome Congress Annual Convention

An event that happens each summer in a different location across the country, it is the largest gathering for those impacted by Down syndrome. Families and self-advocates join together for a weekend of learning and fun. You can register for the convention at their website: *www.ndsccenter.org/register-now*.

National Down Syndrome Awareness Month

October is Down Syndrome Awareness Month, and like WDSD, there are activities and awareness campaigns that spread across the county. For example, New York City's Buddy Walk in Times Square is coordinated every September, as are hundreds of local walks and events across the country. Additionally, an awareness month provides the opportunity for advocates to reach out to their local and national media for educating their community at large about Down syndrome, inclusion, research, and support.

For example, invite your local news agencies to advocacy events, share information relevant to Ds, or alert them to an important life event affecting a person with Down syndrome. These are ways to help educate your community during National Down Syndrome Awareness Month.

Also in October, there is an online and press push for awareness and advocacy. One online event is a challenge hosted by the mom-blogger Michelle Beausoleil Helferich at *http://mdbeau.blogspot.com* called "31 for 21." The challenge is for bloggers within the Ds community to post a blog every day in October in honor of Down Syndrome Awareness Month.

Other Notable National Events

- **321 eConference Education for parents, educators, and advocates in the community.** This tool is celebrated annually over WDSD weekend. The 321 eConference provides online learning whose topics range from potty training to employment to advocacy to the latest research insights.
- **Random Acts of Kindness (RAK)**. In 2015 several U.S. groups gathered to create a logo and spread the word to local groups and individuals to promote RAK on WDSD. The information about the campaign was spread via the national groups involved and their local affiliates. The concept was, "This simple act is sure to spread goodwill and cheer as well as work as an incredible awareness opportunity."
- **DSDN Rockin' Mom Retreat.** This event is for moms only and is a weekend to connect from around the world and participate in service projects for new and expectant parents. You can find out more about it at *www.dsdiagnosisnetwork.org/#!rockin-moms/c1ad4*.
- **International Down Syndrome Coalition Meet Up.** IDSC's yearly meet up for families. This is held at locations across the country for families within the Ds community to gather. *https://theidscorg.presencehost.net/events/idsc-meetup.html*

- **International Mosaic Down Syndrome Association Research and Retreat.** IMDSA hosts a weekend of learning, gathering, and research each year for families connected with mosaic Down syndrome.

Don't forget as well to go to the many local activities that are planned and facilitated around WDSD, October Down Syndrome Awareness Month, and year-round in communities around the world. Check with your local organization or even host your own party.

Blue and Yellow

One thing you will quickly discover during awareness campaigns are the colors blue and yellow. These are widely used in the Ds community. T-shirts, ribbons, bracelets, car decals—lots of visible parts of WDSD and October Awareness Month—employ the blue/yellow theme. So if you are feeling ready to jump in and spread awareness, blue and yellow socks may be a place to start!

Acceptance/Awareness Campaigns

In addition to the UN conference, international and American organizations also arrange awareness campaigns. As your child ages, your advocacy and awareness efforts may change or shift focus; that is just fine! Here are a few campaigns that may be of interest to note as you start out:

Lots of Socks

Down Syndrome International coordinates the "Lots of Socks" awareness campaign to stimulate discussion about Down syndrome. Organizers ask participants to wear unusual or brightly colored socks. When people ask you about your socks, you can explain you're wearing them in honor of people with Down syndrome. You can find out more about the campaign on the WDSD website (*www.worlddown syndromeday.org/lots-of-socks*).

#LifewithDs

In an effort to maintain online awareness of Ds throughout the year, Meriah Nichols, curator of the online community DownSyndrome-Blogs, created the website A Day in the Life with Down Syndrome (*www.adayinthelifewithdownsyndrome.com*), which allows families to share their experiences in a public forum. Participants include families with children of a variety of ages sharing what their everyday living is like. Nichols also uses the hashtag #LifewithDs on Instagram and other social networks to encourage families to post photos they wish to include in the awareness campaign.

Buddy Walks

The Buddy Walk is a fundraising and awareness campaign that largely benefits local Down syndrome affiliates that organize the event. Seven percent of the funds raised are sent to the National Down Syndrome Society, leaving most of the funds to be used locally for programs in the community. The Buddy Walk empowers families to meet other parents in a festive environment and see firsthand the diversity of people with Down syndrome.

Resources

Down Syndrome Facts

- *www.ndsccenter.org/new-and-expectant-parents*
- *www.nichd.nih.gov/health/topics/down/conditioninfo/Pages /risk.aspx*
- *www.dseinternational.org/en-us/about-down-syndrome*

Genetics

- *www.geneticsupportfoundation.org/genetics-and-you/ pregnancy-and-geneticscommon-genetic-conditions-and-birth-defects/chromosome-conditions/down-syndrome*
- *http://learn.genetics.utah.edu/content/chromosomes/diagnose*
- *http://learn.genetics.utah.edu/content/disorders/chromosomal/down*
- *http://ghr.nlm.nih.gov/condition/down-syndrome*

Mosaic Down Syndrome

- *www.IMDSA.org*

Suggested Reading

- "Welcome to Holland": *www.our-kids.org/Archives/Holland.html*

- *What I Should Have Said*: *www.weneedasign.net/#!the-book/cd60*

Finding Local Support

- Down Syndrome Affiliates in Action: *www.dsaia.org/programs/find.html*
- Global Down Syndrome Foundation: *www.globaldownsyndrome.org/about-down-syndrome/resources/local-organizations*
- National Down Syndrome Congress: *www.ndsccenter.org/affiliate-directory*
- National Down Syndrome Society: *www.ndss.org/Resources/Local-Support*

Finding Online Support

- BabyCenter's Down Syndrome Pregnancy Board: *http://community.babycenter.com/groups/a14515/down_syndrome_pregnancy*
- Down Syndrome Diagnosis Network (DSDN): *www.dsdiagnosisnetwork.org*
- International Down Syndrome Coalition (IDSC): *http://theidsc.org/resources/support-for-parents.html*

Chapter Two
A Prenatal Diagnosis

In days past, doctors informed parents their child had Down syndrome at the time of birth. However, with increased access to newer prenatal testing, more expectant mothers are finding out about their child's diagnosis before birth. This can be both empowering and frightening.

Sophisticated as these tests are, the results can sometimes be misleading. Mothers increasingly rely on noninvasive cell-free DNA screening tests such as Harmony, MaterniT21, Panorama, and Verifi to avoid the risk of miscarriage that's associated with diagnostic testing. These cell-free DNA screening tests are done by doing a simple blood test on the pregnant mother, which is completely safe for the baby. DNA segments from the pregnancy can be found in the mother's blood as early as nine weeks' gestation. This test can therefore be done as early as ten weeks' gestation but doctors often wait a few more weeks in order to increase its accuracy. However, all these tests still yield false positives and false negatives. If you receive positive cell-free test results, your doctor should always suggest that you confirm this with a diagnostic test such as an amniocentesis or a chorionic villus sampling. An amniocentesis or "amnio" involves obtaining fetal cells from the maternal amniotic fluid. It is usually done between fifteen and twenty weeks gestation. The chorionic villus sampling or CVS, on the other hand, involves obtaining many fetal cells from the placenta itself. The CVS is usually done between ten to twelve weeks gestation, about a month earlier than the amnio. They are equally accurate; however some doctors feel that the CVS may have a slightly higher risk of causing a miscarriage. Physicians estimate that the risk of the amnio or the CVS causing a pregnancy loss is less than 1 percent.

When your doctor informs you that tests have confirmed your child will be born with Down syndrome, your mind is swirling with thoughts. However, amid all the confusion, remember that this pre-birth diagnosis has given you the gift of time. Your family will have a chance to learn about what life is like with a child with Down syndrome. Your medical team will prepare for a safe delivery. Additionally, a prenatal test result will allow you to tell your loved ones before the birth or at a time of your choosing. This can be a time to celebrate and plan. Read information if that helps you process it all. The most important thing is to prepare for your new child, not a diagnosis.

Prenatal Tests

Throughout your pregnancy, your doctor has taken many opportunities to check on your health and that of your child. This starts in the first trimester and continues until you give birth.

Several of these tests, such as a blood screen or cell-free DNA, will tell you and your doctor if there's a likelihood for a chromosomal anomaly that might indicate Down syndrome. However, it's very important for you to remember that the screening tests only *screen*; the results are not certain, even if results are reported at 99 percent accuracy. When the doctor gets a test result of positive or negative on these screens, that just tells her the probability of a condition such as Down syndrome. Diagnostic tests, such as a CVS or an amniocentesis, as just discussed, provide the greatest accuracy (up to 99 percent), and doctors consider them the only means to determine prior to birth if your child has Down syndrome.

What You Need to Know Before Testing

Before going into a test or a series of tests, there are some things you should think about and some research you should do.

- Begin with the end in mind: Why are you having this testing, and what will you do with the information?
- Understand what tests you are offered (screening versus diagnostic).
- Ask the medical professionals questions about what results each test might yield.
- Satisfy yourself as to whether your physicians will support your decision to move forward.

OUR EXPERIENCE: From a Genetic Counselor

As a genetic counselor, I typically meet with patients following abnormal screening results or abnormal diagnostic testing results during pregnancy. If a screening test indicates an increased risk for Down syndrome, additional testing is offered to confirm the diagnosis. One part of genetic counseling entails candidly discussing the risks, benefits, and complications associated with further testing options. Most patients are understandably highly anxious when they are seen for genetic counseling, regardless of the indication. I work to provide them with the most current and accurate information so they can make the decision that is best for both them and their family. I assure patients that there are no right or wrong emotional responses in this process. When parents receive a new diagnosis of Down syndrome, they are supported in regards to all decisions they consider and ultimately make. One of the best resources I can provide is contact to local families and support groups so they can gain insight into what it's truly like to raise a child with Down syndrome. It can seem overwhelming, but everything will be all right. You are not alone.

—LISA R. JOHNSON, MS, LGC, CERTIFIED GENETIC COUNSELOR

Testing Guidelines

Should you test? It is up to you. Understand what you should know before testing and talk it over with your medical team. In its recommendations for prenatal care, the American Congress of Obstetricians and Gynecologists (ACOG) said in September 2015 that it is now reasonable for all pregnant women, not just women with high-risk pregnancies, to choose cell-free DNA analysis beginning at the 11–14 week appointment. They also recommend that patients are counseled prior to testing (see *www.acog.org/Resources-And-Publications/Committee-Opinions/Committee-on-Genetics/Cell-free-DNA-Screening-for-Fetal-Aneuploidy*).

With the new tests available, the prenatal landscape is changing each year.

Does My Age Matter?

The short answer: Kind of. Advanced maternal age, or AMA, is the clinical term describing pregnant mothers who will be thirty-five or older at the time of delivery. Many people think that most children with Down syndrome are born to mothers in that category. However, since Ds is a genetic condition, it can occur at any age of the mother. A woman's chance of conceiving a child with Down syndrome at the age of thirty is about one in 1,000. At the age of thirty-five, it is about one in 350 and at the age of forty, it is about one in 100. Research by Robert Resta shows that despite women under thirty-five having a lower chance of having a baby with Down syndrome, because those women are a higher percentage of all women giving birth, half of all babies with Down syndrome are *actually* born in women *under* the age of thirty-five. Because a majority of all babies (with Down syndrome or otherwise) are born to women over thirty, the data would naturally suggest that women over thirty are most likely to have a child with Ds. Age factors into the probability of giving birth to a baby with Down syndrome but it is certainly not the only factor.

Screening Tests

Several non-invasive screening tests are available to you during your pregnancy.

During the end of your first trimester (twelve to fourteen weeks gestation), an ultrasound of your baby's neck area, called a nuchal translucency (NT) will often be done in order to determine the probability of your baby having a chromosomal abnormality. Maternal blood tests are also often done at two different occasions in conjunction with this NT ultrasound to help make the results more accurate. The first blood test is done at ten to fourteen weeks gestation, which is at approximately the same time as the NT ultrasound is done. The second one is done at fifteen to twenty weeks gestation. If the NT ultrasound is done with only the first blood test, the Down syndrome detection rate is about 80 percent. If *both* blood tests are done along with the NT ultrasound, the detection rate goes up to 95 percent. It is important to realize that when the detection rate is calculated, the age of the mother is factored in as well, so it is more common for older mothers to have abnormal results and often falsely abnormal results.

More recently, cell-free DNA tests are becoming more popular since they are even more accurate in picking up Down syndrome than these current non-invasive prenatal screening tests, often 99 percent or more. They may also tell you your baby's gender, which is appreciated by many.

It is important to keep in mind that these tests actually test the placenta's DNA, which may not be completely identical to the baby's DNA. There are cases in which the placenta may have some cells with abnormal DNA consistent with Down syndrome (trisomy 21), but the baby itself has normal chromosomes. The only fully accurate tests, therefore, are those that directly use cells from your baby, such as the amnio or CVS.

It is also important to note that the further along you are in your pregnancy, the higher the proportion of placental DNA circulating in the mother's blood, also known as "fetal fraction," so the test may be slightly more reliable if done a little later than nine to ten weeks gestation. In women who are overweight, this may be especially important since they have more maternal DNA fragments in their blood stream and an adequate fetal fraction is often only reached a few weeks later. Talk to your doctor about the best time for you to do this test.

PRENATAL SCREENING TESTS*			
Test	**How It Works**	**When to Test During Pregnancy**	**Results**
Blood Test	Measures the levels of two proteins produced during pregnancy (free Beta-hCG and PAPP-A) via a maternal blood sample	Weeks 9–13	These proteins can indicate a chromosomal issue, such as trisomy 21. Diagnostic testing is necessary for confirming any results.
Ultrasound	Scan evaluates baby's anatomy, specifically looking at: nonvisualized nasal bone, tricuspid regurgitation, crown-rump length, femur and humeral length, head and trunk volume, and umbilical cord diameter. These are considered "soft markers" with none, on their own, being conclusive enough for a recalculation of odds or ever diagnostic. But, they may be considered for suggesting further screening testing	After week 10	The finding, or not finding, of these markers can indicate a chromosomal issue, such as trisomy 21. Diagnostic testing is necessary for confirming any results.
Nuchal Translucency (NT) Test	Measures the clear space in the tissue at the back of baby's neck via an ultrasound	Weeks 11–13	Abnormal levels of these proteins can indicate a chromosomal issue, like trisomy 21. Diagnostic testing is necessary for confirming any results.
Quadruple Screen Test	Measures blood for levels of: AFP, hCG, uE3 and inhibin A via a maternal blood sample	Weeks 15–21	Abnormal levels of these proteins can indicate a chromosomal issue, like trisomy 21. Diagnostic testing is necessary for confirming any results.
Cell-Free DNA Test (Harmony, MaterniT21, Panorama, or Verifi)	Measures placental DNA in the mother's blood via a maternal blood sample. Accuracy of these tests increases along with the length of the pregnancy.	After week 10	Detects certain genetic conditions. Diagnostic testing is necessary for confirming any results.

*Accuracy of these tests increases along with the length of the pregnancy. Analysis of baby's DNA to detect certain genetic conditions. Diagnostic testing is necessary for confirming any results.

Source: *http://americanpregnancy.org/prenatal-testing*

View a text version of this table

What Do My Screening Results Mean?

If you have undergone a screening test, the results you receive may be confusing. Start with the most important point: *A "positive" screen is not a positive diagnosis*, even if it touts 99 percent accuracy.

Data from the screen, along with other information such as your age, are factored together to provide the probability of the baby having Down syndrome. Unless you have a diagnostic test, like a CVS or an amniocentesis, the positive result only means that you have a greater likelihood of having a child with Ds. Be sure to ask your genetic counselor or physician to help you understand your results. As we said earlier, the only way to know with 99 percent accuracy whether your child will have Ds is through a diagnostic test.

OUR EXPERIENCE: Prenatal Screenings

At eighteen weeks our quad screen came back with an increased risk of our baby having Down syndrome. We went for a level-2 ultrasound and learned that our baby girl had a condition called ventriculomegaly and shortened long bones in her arms and legs. While this was not a significant factor, her shortened long bones increased our chances of Down syndrome to fifty-fifty. Two weeks later, we returned for another ultrasound in which a heart defect was discovered, further increasing our odds.

We refused to risk our pregnancy by performing an amniocentesis, and noninvasive maternal-fetal blood tests were very new to the market. Ultimately, we fully accepted the fact that we would wait another eighteen-plus weeks to know, for sure, whether our daughter would be born with Down syndrome. At thirty-seven weeks, our beautiful, amazing daughter Ellie was born and just so happened to have Down syndrome, just as all of the ultrasounds had indicated. We have no regrets having chosen to "wait it out." Our medical follow-ups and routine ultrasounds were enough for us to know what we were to expect medically upon her birth, and her having Down syndrome was an afterthought.

—AARON AND LAUREN OCHALEK

Ultrasound Markers

You may find out there is a chance your baby could have Down syndrome during an ultrasound. There are several markers that the sonographer may note during your anatomy scan. Remember: *These are not diagnostic*. They don't absolutely mean your baby has Ds. Often, babies with typical chromosomes have one or more of these markers. (It is also possible that your baby might have Down syndrome and not have any of these markers during pregnancy at all.) If the doctor notes markers, she may recommend further testing.

Markers may include:

- Echogenic intracardiac focus (EIF)—a bright spot on the heart
- Mild pyelectasis—enlargement of the kidney
- Single umbilical artery (SUA)—one artery on the umbilical cord, rather than two
- Echogenic bowel—a bright spot on bowel
- Cerebral ventriculomegaly/hydrocephalus—*the brain* is surrounded by a clear fluid
- Choroid plexus cysts (CPCs)—there are fluid-filled spaces in the brain

- Enlarged cisterna magna—there is a space between two parts of the brain
- Fifth finger clinodactyly—the baby has a curved pinkie finger
- Short femur length—leg bone(s) measure behind the baby's other measurements
- Short humerus length—arm bone(s) measure behind the baby's other measurements
- Thickened nuchal fold—increased fluid at the back of the baby's neck
- Nasal Bone—shortened or absent nasal bone

Source: *http://sogc.org/wp-content/uploads/2013/01/162E-CPG-June20051.pdf*

OUR EXPERIENCE: Ultrasounds

We had an increased nuchal fold, absent nasal bone, short femur, and kidney issue at our nineteen-week scan. Down syndrome was confirmed through amnio at twenty-three weeks.

—KARI REICHMUTH

Normal nuchal folds, normal femur length, normal humerus bone length, no heart defects seen, but always two weeks behind in gestation date.

—CILLA BISHELL

Quad screen showed elevated risk, so we went for a level-2 ultrasound at eighteen weeks. That showed shortened long bones in the arms and legs. Our OB was concerned and about a month later checked the blood flow through the cord, which was abnormal so we started doing growth scans and they finally found her heart defect (Atrioventricular Septal Defect—AVSD) at the thirty-one-week scan. It had been missed in at least four ultrasounds before that.

—MELISSA MOOS

I had no markers and was also told they saw all four chambers of his heart. Boy, were they wrong! He was born with a complete AVSD.

—KHOURY SHAKOFSKY

No markers at all, and I had four ultrasounds altogether.

—MEGAN

We couldn't get a good picture of the nasal bone at twenty weeks. I had another scan at twenty-two weeks and they found it. No markers for T21—didn't even see the Atrioventricular (AV) canal defect.

—ANDREA WINKLER

I had ultrasounds every couple weeks due to being high risk due to a bleeding disorder. We did not have one marker. She was actually measuring bigger due to her long femurs.

—JESSY POWERS

At my twenty-week scan there was extra fluid around the kidneys, but no one was too worried as it was "common at that stage." We repeated eight weeks later, and everything was how it should be. However, at around thirty-six weeks I had a third ultrasound done, and even then you couldn't see any markers physically.

—BRIANNA LARDIE

Diagnostic Tests

Some of you may choose to do a diagnostic test so you can have an answer before your child is born. Often you'll decide on this course of action because a screening indicates your baby is at an increased risk, and your medical team recommends a more definitive testing option. In comparison to the screenings, diagnostic tests provide information about whether the baby has a genetic condition. The test is based on cell analysis and is 99 percent accurate. Because these tests are more invasive, though, there is a risk of miscarriage.

PRENATAL DIAGNOSTIC TESTS			
Test	**How It Works**	**When to Test During Pregnancy**	**Results**
Chorionic Villus Sampling (CVS)	Placental DNA (which may share the baby's genetic material) is collected during an office procedure.	Weeks 10–13	Up to 99 percent in determining chromosomal conditions, like trisomy 21. Preliminary results can take a few days. Full results can take up to a few weeks.
Amniocentesis (Amnio)	Amniotic fluid (which contains placental DNA) is collected through a needle. An ultrasound is used to guide the collection.	After week 14	Up to 99 percent in determining chromosomal conditions, like trisomy 21. Preliminary results, like the fluorescence in situ hybridization (FISH), might be available in a few days and look for specific information. Full results can take up to a few weeks.

Source: *http://americanpregnancy.org/prenatal-testing*

View a text version of this table

OUR EXPERIENCE: On Having Diagnostic Prenatal Testing

When the doctors found a larger nuchal fold and swollen ventricles in her brain at my twenty-week ultrasound, we were then scheduled for a more in-depth ultrasound. They found a small nasal bone, and our odds of the baby having Down syndrome were one in eight. Doing the amnio was a struggle for us. When they originally told us about the risk of miscarriage, we said no to the amnio, but when our chances came back so high, we needed to know for sure. It came down to me *having* to know one way or another so I could prepare. I'm so glad we did the test. I grieved *really* hard when we got the positive result, but by the time she was born I was in a much better place and I could connect and enjoy her. Also, if we wouldn't have gotten the Ds diagnosis, they wouldn't have sent us for a heart echo where they found her heart defects. That allowed us to choose the right hospital and have the resources to do surgery if she needed it immediately. I believe it saved her life!

—BRENDA HICKSON

During our twenty-week anatomy scan, there were several markers including a shortened femur and smaller head size. A week later, we had another ultrasound at a specialized clinic that showed basically the same thing and a choroid plexus cyst in the brain. We were told the cysts were typically inconsequential but are more common in a child with a trisomy. Afterward, we met the genetics counselor and were given lots of numbers and probabilities. I was just twenty-five years old at conception, so the chance that our child would be born with trisomy 21 was minute. The risk of complication from an amniocentesis was higher. We declined the amniocentesis. We opted for closer monitoring to ensure that if the baby had a trisomy, we could catch any organ anomalies and be prepared. Following an ultrasound at thirty-four weeks that showed a more round head shape, we opted for an amniocentesis to give a definite answer. The risks were less severe to the baby at that point. We told ourselves that the outcome didn't matter, but it was a long weekend waiting for the results. On Monday, I called the genetics counselor. Our child did indeed have forty-seven chromosomes.

—JENNY DHEIN

Receiving Your Prenatal Diagnosis

After undergoing prenatal testing, your biggest challenge will be waiting for the results. In 2009 Dr. Brian Skotko and his team, and in 2011 Kathryn Sheets of the National Society of Genetic Counselors, laid out guidelines for how the diagnosis should be presented to families. It was determined that a medical professional should deliver the results:

- Through the health-care provider most knowledgeable about Ds
- To both parents, together
- During a personal visit, rather than a phone call or written correspondence
- Using sensitive, neutral language
- Along with up-to-date, accurate information and resources on life with Down syndrome

If you feel your medical team did not deliver the news appropriately, sharing these guidelines with them may change how they deliver a diagnosis in the future. There are groups that can help, such as your local DSA, which may do educational outreach to medical professionals in your area, and DSDN, which can help you craft a feedback letter to your medical team. See *www.brianskotko.com* and *http://obgyn.duke.edu/sites/obgyn.duke.edu/files/NSGCPracticeGuidelinesCommunicatingDiagnosisDS_0.pdf* for the guidelines.

OUR EXPERIENCE: Hearing the News

We chose prenatal testing because of the high risk of trisomy with our fourth pregnancy. I was forty-one, and our first pregnancies had ended in miscarriages. We knew that at least two of those were caused by trisomies, so we were high-risk. My OB/GYN recommended the Harmony blood test, which I took at ten weeks. It was a simple blood draw, followed by a two-week wait. I was grateful for the early peace of mind the test would give me, no matter what the result—and I was excited to learn the gender that early. When our test came back, we were told it was with a 99.9 percent positive chance of T21. I was devastated at first. Although the test was not diagnostic, we prepared as if our son had Down syndrome. With the time to prepare, learn, and build a support community, I found my way back to joy long before our little bundle was born. When he arrived, it was all thrill and no grief, all celebration and no shock. I'm so grateful I had the time to process the news with my husband, family, and friends in advance—without the risky amniocentesis process.

—ERIC AND BECKY BAUSMAN

Now What?

It can take a few minutes, hours, days, or weeks for the information to really soak in. Seek out medical professionals who will support you. Give yourself time to process all of the information. Find a local Down syndrome organization so you can talk with parents. Join online communities through organizations such as the Down Syndrome Diagnosis Network or BabyCenter's Down Syndrome Pregnancy (you will find both in the resources section) to meet other parents with a new diagnosis.

Processing a Diagnosis

Parents report a wide variety of emotions when hearing about their child's diagnosis. For most, this is news that you never expected to hear. For many of you, Down syndrome is a condition that you know very little about. You may well find a level of acceptance as your child's due date draws near. While the path to acceptance is personal, many of your stories are similar.

OUR EXPERIENCE: Are You Glad You Knew?

Truthfully I was glad I knew, and it was okay. I knew I could do this. [The doctors] thought it was trisomy 13 or 18, and I was just relieved that the baby did not have one of them. I didn't even cry at the news.

—JENNIFER WINTERS

The first moments were the hardest. Lots of thoughts racing through my mind. By the time the test results came back, I was ready to just move forward and meet my baby.

—JENNY

I wish that we wouldn't have found out. Too much time was spent worrying and researching when we should have just been enjoying the pregnancy.

—TANYA

I am so glad I knew. I was able to deal with all of my emotions prior to his birth, and was able to actually celebrate and rejoice when he finally arrived. We were told it was a little girl. We were overjoyed!

—SHANNON BERRY

We did the first trimester screen because we wanted to be prepared, and we loved seeing our baby during the ultrasound. Three markers pointed to a chromosomal abnormality: an increased nuchal fold, an echogenic intracardiac focus, and a missing nasal bone. I cried through the rest of the appointment. We were not prepared for this diagnosis and did the Harmony test. The first days were a blur, full of every possible emotion: I was sad, angry, disappointed, scared, [and] felt helpless and hopeless. I kept asking the same question: Why us?

We considered termination but at the same time couldn't imagine killing our child. An amniocentesis confirmed the Harmony results. Around the same time, we learned about Targeted Nutritional Intervention, which we believe addresses the metabolic imbalances resulting from the extra chromosome. We were relieved to learn that we could help our daughter. A few weeks later, an echocardiogram showed a congenital heart defect. We had just adjusted to the diagnosis, but now thought about termination again. We worried about our firstborn, whom we didn't want to suffer. Two weeks later, our baby was given only a 50 percent survival chance. Termination came up again, and I remember the desperate feeling of just wanting this baby out of my body. It's heartbreaking to have a choice. Life has been exhausting, but every smile rewards us. There would be a big hole in our life and in my heart if she wasn't here.

—PEET BUCHANAN

Pregnancy Monitoring

Once a diagnosis is suspected or the physician has confirmed your child has Down syndrome, there are medical care considerations for the remainder of your pregnancy. Because the rate of pregnancy loss is sometimes higher with a trisomy, you and your medical team will be proactive in monitoring the baby, especially as the due date draws near.

Choosing a Medical Team

Having physicians and specialists who share your values and beliefs will be critical in the remainder of your pregnancy. Additionally, you may now be considered a high-risk pregnancy and be referred to a specialist. A maternal-fetal medicine (MFM) physician or perinatologist specializes in the care of women and babies who fall into a higher risk category. Talk with your primary-care provider or OB/GYN about whether your pregnancy should be monitored by a specialist. Consider speaking with a genetic counselor (GC) to have your questions answered and gain a better understanding of Down syndrome. The GC will be able to provide many resources and information specific to your needs.

Questions to Consider about Your Medical Team

- Have they been supportive of you as a patient in the past?
- Do they have the proper training that you might need?
- Do you feel they delivered the diagnosis appropriately?
- Can you count on them to handle your care most effectively and seek out specialists for anything that might come up?

OUR EXPERIENCE: Choosing Medical Care

When we received an increased risk for our daughter having Down syndrome, I decided to switch to a different OB and pediatric clinic. After receiving the diagnosis in a negative way, I wanted to be sure that the [new] doctor would support me. I also wanted to be sure that the doctors were more familiar with high-risk pregnancies and infants with special needs. I asked my maternal-fetal medicine specialist for OB recommendations and I contacted our local Ds organization about finding a pediatrician. The process was relatively easy. It required a few phone calls and I went to an orientation at the pediatric clinic to check it out. The time spent was well worth it to have doctors who I feel support my family.

—ANGELA DEWISPELAERE

Prenatal Care with a Down Syndrome Diagnosis

As we mentioned earlier, there is sometimes an increased risk for pregnancy loss when a baby has trisomy 21. To ensure you have a safe delivery, the American Congress of Obstetricians and Gynecologists (ACOG) recommends additional monitoring precautions. Although there is not a standardized care plan, medical teams will evaluate your pregnancy along the way and may use some of the following tools to determine care for you and your child.

Ultrasound Exam

During the pregnancy, your OB/GYN will usually perform at least one level-2 ultrasound scan. She will look for anatomical features and determine any concerns that may need to be addressed during pregnancy or after birth. Sonographers will examine and measure the baby and look closely at the heart and intestines and monitor growth. These scans are important, since some conditions are more prevalent in babies with Down syndrome. For example, there's a condition of the intestine, duodenal atresia or a "double bubble," that requires surgery after birth. It can be seen via ultrasound in the second and third trimester. The doctor may repeat ultrasounds several times as a way to check the health of your baby.

Non-Stress Test (NST)

An NST is a noninvasive test that monitors your baby's heart rate and possible contractions via a belt on your abdomen. During the test, technicians record and evaluate your baby's heart rate. This test is recommended after twenty-eight weeks. A physician will typically schedule rounds of NSTs closer to the end of pregnancy as another way to monitor the baby.

Biophysical Profile (BPP)

Your doctor may well want to do a biophysical profile, a specialized ultrasound that examines the welfare of your baby during pregnancy. The baby is evaluated in five ways, including: heart rate, muscle tone, breathing movement, movements, and amniotic fluid volume. During this ultrasound, the technician gives each of those five areas a score from 0–2 to calculate the total score. According to ACOG, a score of 8–10 is reassuring in terms of the baby's welfare. If the baby scores a 6, more information is needed for comparison, and a BPP is usually repeated within twenty-four hours, depending on how far along the pregnancy is. A score of 4 or below indicates a need for more information quickly and might mean that you're about to give birth.

Fetal Echocardiogram

Because up to 50 percent of children with Down syndrome may have a heart defect, your doctor should review the baby's heart during your pregnancy and shortly after birth. This test will allow you and your medical staff to prepare for what needs your baby will have. Conditions that an echocardiogram may reveal are:

- Atrioventricular canal defect
- Ventricular septal defect
- Atrial septal defect
- Patent ductus arteriosus
- Tetralogy of Fallot

If one or more of these concerns are seen, a cardiologist will join your medical team. Your team will provide you with information about the defect, how it will be managed/treated, and whether your child will need surgery to correct it. The success rate for heart repair is very high.

Doppler Ultrasound of the Umbilical Artery

Another area physicians may monitor is the umbilical artery. Using an ultrasound scan, they'll examine the cord blood flow in the placenta. If it's too low, it can mean that there is a decrease in the amount of oxygen being delivered to the baby.

Fetal Kick Count

The baby should kick and move regularly by the third trimester. Because of the increased risk of stillbirth in a trisomy pregnancy, it is important for you to be proactive and aware of your baby's movement. Time how long it takes you to feel ten movements (including kicks, rolls, and flutters). You should feel these movements in less than two hours. If you have counted for two blocks of time without at least ten movements or if the movements have not followed your typical pattern, you should contact your physician.

NOTE FROM THE AUTHOR

After a "positive" screen on the verifi test, my doctors laid out a plan for prenatal care for the remaining half of my pregnancy. We scheduled a level-2 ultrasound that would take a closer look at the baby. A fetal echocardiogram was scheduled to check over the heart again. During that scan, the doctors discovered pericardial effusion (fluid around the heart) so they began to monitor his heart more closely.

As the due date got closer and weekly appointments began, I visited the doctor twice a week—once to the OB and once to the perinatologist. The OB monitored me and performed NSTs each week. The perinatologist did the ultrasound and BPP each week and looked at the blood flow from the umbilical cord. My doctors shared the data they collected, and I monitored the baby's movements through kick counts. One week before my due date, we all made the decision to induce because the heart fluid was increasing. It was very comforting throughout my pregnancy to have specialists monitoring us. The extra care helped me to stay calm and remember the joy that comes with pregnancy too.

—Jen

When You Need to Talk

Several areas have followed the lead of Massachusetts and established a First Call program for parents of children with Down syndrome. The Massachusetts Down Syndrome Congress (MDSC) provides a twenty-four-hour phone service for parents with a new diagnosis who would like to talk with someone. The parent-mentoring program offers callers peer support, as well as accurate information and connections to resources. "Parents First Call is the heart and soul of our organization," says Sarah Cullen, Family Support Director of MDSC. "Receiving accurate, up-to-date information and the opportunity to connect with a parent who has traveled a similar journey is invaluable. Knowing that you are not alone and feeling a sense of community and hope is priceless." Check out the details at *www.mdsc.org/programs/ParentsFirstCall.cfm*. To find out if your area offers this service, contact your local Ds organization or area hospital.

Sharing the News

Some families choose to share with others the moment that Down syndrome is suspected, whether in pregnancy or shortly after birth. Here are some key points to remember when sharing the news.

- **Set the Tone**—It was a challenge to have such mixed emotions while trying to also lead a "normal" life. It proved especially challenging as a very noticeably pregnant woman, as this becomes a source of small talk with everyone until delivery. I found that when I was struggling to come to terms with the diagnosis and talked with people about it, their responses were mostly negative. That is when I had the sad faces and "I'm sorrys." As I grew to accept the diagnosis and share with others, reactions and responses were much more understanding and positive. Sharing the news and setting a positive tone in conversation helped others respond accordingly.

- **Respect Their Process**—Each person will respond differently to your news. Close family and friends may not share your feelings and need to work through their own. Give everyone time and connect when they're ready.
- **Provide Them with Resources**—Many of your friends and family will have little background knowledge to draw from about Down syndrome. By giving connections to books and links to resources, you will help build your support team.
- **Share When *You* Are Ready**—The "right" time to share is different for everyone. If you can, discuss it with your spouse or partner. Consider your feelings and make the right choice for your family.

OUR EXPERIENCE: How We Shared the News

We wanted his birth met with only joy. No speculation or surprises. We told people not long before he was born because he was two months early. We posted notes on Facebook and sent e-mails to family and friends. There was no room for "Sorry," and only congratulations were said.

—MELISSA CHAMBERS

We told our families and a handful of close friends right after we found out (via amnio). I plan on making a larger Facebook announcement once he's born; I just felt like I really wanted to introduce him to the world with his name first—not his diagnosis. Everyone that we have told has been *extremely* supportive. I knew this pregnancy would be a lot more stressful, and I honestly just wanted everyone else to be positive and happy and not feel awkward about what to say to me.

—EMILY PELTON

Yes! We just wanted those that love us to know what we knew about our daughter. We didn't feel like Down syndrome was a secret or anything that needed hiding. We also wanted people to be able to educate themselves.

—TARA BARNES

I wanted the support of friends and family. And I wanted her birth to be a happy occasion for everyone and not a disappointment. I didn't want a bunch of pity looks and "I'm sorry."

—HEATHER HOLBROOK

From the Authors of *Diagnosis to Delivery: A Pregnant Mother's Guide to Down Syndrome*

After supporting pregnant moms for more than five years on the BabyCenter Down Syndrome Pregnancy board, we found some questions regularly bubbled to the surface—like how to deal with insensitive comments, how to share the news, how to deal with medical issues, and how to prepare brothers and sisters. Expectant parents had some concerns and perspectives that were different from the material normally covered in new parent books. Because we found these kinds of questions arising so often, we felt it would be helpful to create a book that could consistently provide those answers with different layers of support.

—Stephanie Meredith and Nancy Iannone

A Sample Letter for Sharing the News

In their book *Diagnosis to Delivery: A Pregnant Mother's Guide to Down Syndrome*, Stephanie Meredith and Nancy Iannone offer a sample e-mail to loved ones telling them that the baby has Down syndrome.

OUR EXPERIENCE: Dear Friends and Family,

Hello and I hope this e-mail finds you all well. As you all know, we are expecting our baby on [due date]. We have learned that the baby is a [boy or girl], and we have named [him or her] [his or her name]. We are so very excited about this addition to our family. (Add any personalized details you want to share.)

We have recently learned that our sweet baby has Down syndrome (and whatever ancillary issues if any). We learned the results through a genetic test called [an amniocentesis or a CVS], which is virtually 100 percent accurate (and the testing that revealed the ancillary issues, such as an echocardiogram).

Of course this news has left us overwhelmed. We are still adjusting. If you see us, we may still be showing signs of shock, but we have learned from other parents that we will move away from this time of turmoil to a place of excitement and amazement. One thing we know for sure: we love our baby [boy or girl], and we hope you will join us in welcoming [him or her].

We know that you must have many questions, and we will try our best to answer, but we have a lot to learn in the next few months about Down syndrome. We have already started to research, and you can look at DownSyndromePregnancy.org for some basic information for friends and family. They even have a booklet just for you, *Your Loved One Is Having a Baby with Down Syndrome.* Some of the most important things we have learned are that each person with Down syndrome is a unique individual, and that recent advances in medicine, education, and acceptance have greatly improved the lives of people with Down syndrome. More importantly, we have learned that our [son or daughter] will live a rich and rewarding life, and will enrich ours as well.

We know many of you may not know what to say to us when you see us—and we understand. We're not sure we would have known what to say either. We would appreciate if you could avoid saying, "I'm sorry." We have heard from other parents that they hear this a lot, and it tends to hurt after a while. We have listed a few websites that might help.

We will keep you updated about any issues that come up and when little [name] arrives. Thank you all so much for your love for us and for welcoming our little one.

With love,

[Your signature]

Websites:

NDSS (National Down Syndrome Society)

NDSC (National Down Syndrome Congress)

Down Syndrome Online (by DownsEd)

LuMind Research Down Syndrome Foundation

Down Syndrome Diagnosis Network

Stone Soup "What to say" (A helpful blog post)

Reprinted with permission: Down Syndrome Pregnancy *http://downsyndromepregnancy.org* which also includes a newborn book, a pregnancy book, and relatives book, as well as articles for new and expectant parents.

OUR EXPERIENCE: Looking Back: Delivering after a Diagnosis

When we received the diagnosis, I felt like my life was over. It was like being in a fog, like I was surrounded by this darkness I had to try to grope my way out of. And no one could help, because no one else could understand. No one I knew had a child with Down syndrome. My family and friends were sympathetic, and they tried to say the right things, but really, what are the right things? I'm still not really sure.

Of course, the fog slowly lifted. After weeks of crying and grieving, acceptance slowly came. I gathered the strength to start learning about Down syndrome and about what I would need to do. I came to realize that many of the fears I had were based on extremely outdated misconceptions and stereotypes. Medical advances, early intervention programs, and resources have allowed people with Down syndrome to do more than they ever had before. By the time Wyatt was born, I was at peace with who he was. I could be happy welcoming him into the world, extra chromosome and all.

With Wyatt now fifteen months old, I can say this with confidence: raising a child with Down syndrome is not that different from raising a "normal" child. They're babies first. They need to be changed, and fed, and loved. That's about it. Day to day, I don't really think much about Down syndrome at all. It isn't something that has much of an effect on our lives, really. We were blessed in that Wyatt doesn't have any major health problems, so he's never had to go on any kind of special medications or undergo surgery. He likes music, he babbles to himself in the car, and he loves to cuddle with his mama. He's a normal baby. Raising a child with Down syndrome does not doom you to a life of misery and sadness and despair, but neither does it grant you a life of awesome sunshine and daisies and rainbows. My life isn't any fuller with love because of Down syndrome than it was without it. There's more love because Wyatt is my child—not because he has an extra chromosome.

—CASSY FIANO CHESSER

Resources

Online Resources

- DownSyndromePregnancy.org (includes the booklet *Your Loved One Is Having a Baby with Down Syndrome*): *http://downsyndromepregnancy.org*
- National Down Syndrome Society (NDSS): *www.ndss.org*
- National Down Syndrome Congress (NDSC): *www.ndsccenter.org*
- Down Syndrome Education Online (by DownsEd): *www.down-syndrome.org*
- LuMind Research Down Syndrome Foundation: *www.lumindfoundation.org*
- Down Syndrome Diagnosis Network: *www.dsdiagnosisnetwork.org*
- Stone Soup "What to Say" (A helpful blog post) *https://katrinastonoff.wordpress.com/2007/10/09/what-to-say-when-your-friends-baby-has-down-syndrome/*
- Down Syndrome Pregnancy (*http://downsyndromepregnancy.org*), which also includes a newborn book, a pregnancy book, and relatives book, as well as articles for new and expectant parents. Reprinted with permission.
- BabyCenter's Down Syndrome Pregnancy Board: *http://community.babycenter.com/groups/a14515/down_syn*

drome_pregnancy

- International Down Syndrome Coalition (IDSC): *http://theidsc.org/resources/support-for-parents.html*

Finding Information about Down Syndrome

- American College of Obstetrics and Gynecologists: *www.acog.org/-/media/For-Patients/faq133.pdf?dmc=1&ts=20150506T1318221347*
- Down Syndrome Prenatal Testing: *www.downsyndromeprenataltesting.com*
- National Center for Prenatal and Postnatal Down Syndrome Resources: *http://downsyndromediagnosis.org*
- National Society of Genetic Counselors: *http://obgyn.duke.edu/sites/obgyn.duke.edu/files/NSGCPracticeGuidelinesCommunicatingDiagnosisDS.pdf*

Finding Local Support

- Down Syndrome Affiliates in Action: *www.dsaia.org/programs/find.html*
- Global Down Syndrome Foundation: *www.globaldownsyndrome.org/about-down-syndrome/resources/local-organizations*
- National Down Syndrome Congress: *www.ndsccenter.org/affiliate-directory*
- National Down Syndrome Society: *www.ndss.org/Resources/Local-Support*
- Genetic Support Foundation: *www.geneticsupportfoundation.org/genetics-and-*

you/pregnancy-and-genetics/common-genetic-conditions-and-birth-defects/chromosome-conditions/down-syndrome

Suggested Reading

- Beck, Martha. *Expecting Adam: A True Story of Birth, Rebirth, and Everyday Magic*. New York: Berkley Publishing Group, 2000.
- Jacob, Jennifer. *Unexpected: Stories of a Down Syndrome Diagnosis*. *www.missiont21.com*.
- Nichols, Meriah. *Expecting a Child with Down Syndrome*. *www.meriahnichols.com/expecting-a-child-with-down-syndrome*.
- Soper, K. *Gifts: Mothers Reflect on How Children with Down Syndrome Enrich Their Lives*. Bethesda, MD: Woodbine House, 2007.

Chapter Three
A Birth Diagnosis

The birth of a child typically evokes feelings of joy, excitement, and celebration. For many families whose babies receive a birth diagnosis of Down syndrome, the emotions can also include sadness, confusion, and fear. There is no right or wrong reaction. The baby you have prepared for so diligently is not at all what you expected. You may feel bewildered. You may have feelings of grief, confusion, and worry, yet your love for that baby—*your* baby—is incredibly real and as strong as any bond between a parent and child.

At first, every second is filled with new thoughts, feelings, and fears. What will your baby's life be like as she or he grows up? How will you handle the increased responsibility that comes with having a child with special needs? Perhaps most poignant, how will the arrival of this baby, with its unexpected extra needs, affect your other children? But those first confusing, terrifying seconds turn to minutes, then to hours, and finally to days and months passing with your baby. You are smiling again. Your baby is smiling, cooing and snuggling, and bonding with your other children—and them with him or her. You realize that your baby is just that: a baby, more alike than different in so many beautiful ways. Down syndrome is now a part of your life, but it has not become your life.

Diagnosis at Birth

Shortly after your child is born, medical staff and/or you may notice indicators for Down syndrome. Just because a baby may have a few of these markers does not necessarily mean she has Down syndrome. The only way to determine a diagnosis is through blood testing and analysis of your baby's chromosomes, called a karyotype, which will take up to a few weeks. Waiting for results can be a very challenging time and can be magnified if other concerns arise. It is important to listen and ask questions and to spend time getting to know your baby. This may not be a diagnosis you were expecting, but your baby needs you just the same. When looking at your child, you may notice some characteristics of Down syndrome, but look for the family features that are sure to be there, as well. Although your child may have an extra chromosome, she is still very much a part of you.

Common Physical Attributes of Those with Down Syndrome

- Decreased or poor muscle tone (hypotonia)
- Short neck, with excess skin at the back of the neck
- Flattened facial profile and nose
- Small head, ears, and mouth
- Upward slanting eyes, often with a skin fold that comes out from the upper eyelid and covers the inner corner of the eye (epicanthal folds)
- White spots on the colored part of the eye (Brushfield spots)
- Wide, short hands with short fingers
- A single, deep crease across the palm of the hand (palmar crease)
- A deep groove between the first and second toes (sandal toe gap)

OUR EXPERIENCE: Waiting on a Diagnosis

From Mom: When the pediatrician told us he suspected our son had Down syndrome, we were shocked. He couldn't be sure either way, wouldn't give us any odds, and told us we would have to wait four days for the karyotype. I didn't know how much to research or allow myself to think my son might have it. I would stare at him and try to tell if I could "see it" or not. I felt so in limbo. I cried when I felt overwhelmed with the possibility of a life with Ds, then forced myself to push it out of my mind because he might not have it. My husband refused to consider the possibility until the results were in, so I felt alone in trying to process what was going on. Everyone knew he was born and wanted to visit or call. We didn't share the suspicion beyond immediate family members, so I didn't know what to say. I didn't want any visitors because I was so emotional. I should have been so happy celebrating the birth of my son, but I felt so much sadness and fear over the unknown. I felt robbed of that priceless time with my son and my family.

From Dad: Less than an hour after our son was born, our family was turned upside down with questions but no answers. That was after the pediatrician told us that he "suspected" Down syndrome in our son but wasn't certain. We'd have to wait for confirmation from genetic testing; [the wait was] four days. In the meantime, we were left to sort through the emotions, which went from jovial to confused to sadness to denial. I refused to accept the diagnosis until it could be proven true. Why focus on something if it wasn't entirely clear? That didn't work as the wait became agonizing and emotional, checking his hands for the crease, his toes for the gap. Is there anything that can clearly tell us what is going on? The wait was tougher than the initial diagnosis. What does this mean for our family? Four days, really?

—NICK AND JENNY DI BENEDETTO

Advice for Families

Having a birth diagnosis can feel like a very traumatic time in your life. You have waited so long for your little one and are thankful to have safely delivered him. Then you may notice something from those in the room—a look, a whisper—that causes you to pause and wonder. It is important to be kind to yourself and take one day at a time. Lean on the support system you have in place, seek out local organizations and families in your area, and find professionals to guide you through. You may be ready to reach out the first day, or you may not be ready for months. Move forward on your own timeline; just know there are many resources available to help you navigate it all.

OUR EXPERIENCE: A Near-Certain Diagnosis

From Mom: This was finally the beginning of my much-anticipated labor to deliver my eighth child, our fourth girl. My labor progressed quickly, and in a few hours I was ready to push. Three strong pushes and Brianna Joy was placed on the outside of my belly. The moment I saw her, I knew. There was something very unfamiliar about her. She was crying, and her eyes were tightly squinted and slanting upward, her head was noticeably smaller, and she had very tiny ears. Also, her skin tone had a very purple hue (which later would be attributed to the significant heart defect she had kept hidden in utero despite several sonograms). My immediate thought was, "Oh wow, she has Down syndrome." I really knew very little about Ds, and it was not a concern of mine at all throughout my pregnancy, despite the fact that at forty-five, I was of "advanced maternal age" and supposedly at "risk" for chromosomal anomalies. I just knew in the flurry of the post-birth activities going on around me that our lives had changed forever.

From Dad: [I was a physician and had] delivered our past three children. The birth process progressed as had our previous experiences. Little Brianna came into the world surrounded by the usual fanfare—and relief—of all in the room. And then, as one awakening from a very real, deep, involved dream, things began to change. My first realization that something wasn't "normal" was the tone in my wife's voice as she asked whether the baby was okay. Thinking medically, I had no reason, no symptom, no change in vital signs to think otherwise so I reassured her all was well. And then the follow-up, concern-laden persistence of my soulmate commanded attention. Looking closely at the little girl in her arms revealed little slanted eyes, an unusually round face, and little palms with the trademark crease of Down syndrome. One look into the attending nurse's eyes confirmed this diagnosis and life as we knew it changed forever.

—DR. STEVE AND JOY GRIFFIN

Receiving a Birth Diagnosis

When a Down syndrome diagnosis is suspected at birth, it is important that your family receives the news in an appropriate way. Emotions are high, and there may be medical factors, such as breathing, heart or body temperature concerns, that take precedence over the suspected diagnosis. The American Academy of Pediatrics reminds its physicians to first offer words of congratulations to the parents on the birth of the new child. Beginning with a focus on your baby sets a positive tone for an often-difficult conversation. We suggest you refer to the previous chapter for the specific guidelines that were laid out by Dr. Brian Skotko and his team in 2009 and by Kathryn Sheets et al. for the National Society of Genetic Counselors in 2011.

Where to Turn for Information

There are many resources to help support a family new to the Ds community. One of the best places to begin is your local Down syndrome organization, if you have one. Finding people in your community to lean on for support, information, and advice can be very helpful. For a list of Ds organizations across the country, visit the Global Down Syndrome Foundation, Down Syndrome Affiliates in Action, or the NDSS websites to find groups near you. If you are not near a local organization, contact the Down Syndrome Diagnosis Network (DSDN). They will help to find you connections with other parents in your area.

Confirming a Diagnosis

Once your physician suspects your baby has Down syndrome, the only way to confirm this is through an analysis of the baby's DNA. Before your child leaves the hospital, a blood sample will be taken and sent to a lab for testing. The testing will produce a karyotype, which enables physicians to examine the number of chromosomes and any structural changes within them. It can take up to two weeks for full results. A genetic counselor can help you understand and interpret the results; if you don't wish to consult one, your physician will play this role.

Should I Meet with a Genetic Counselor?

After receiving the diagnosis, you may be offered an appointment to talk with a genetic counselor (GC) to discuss the implications. You may find it helpful to learn more about Ds and for information on which type your child has. The GC will also discuss what having a child with a trisomy means for your current or future children and may suggest additional testing for you and your partner. A GC will also have resources for you as a parent and will be able to answer many questions that you and your family have.

Processing a Diagnosis

Like any new information that catches you off-guard, a child's diagnosis can be quite a shock. Many months of preparing and dreaming about the baby about to enter your life are flipped upside down with a few words. A post-birth diagnosis carries a wide range of emotions and responses. None are right or wrong; they are yours.

Take each day as it comes and try to be in the moment with your child.

OUR EXPERIENCE: Hearing the Diagnosis

We welcomed Alvaro into the world at thirty-seven weeks. It was magical. Four hours after he was born, the magical feelings were crushed. The pediatrician asked everyone to leave the room. She began to explain that she believed he had Down syndrome. She shared the markers that led to her suspicions: the low muscle tone, the slanted eyes, and the crease across the palm in his hand. I felt as if the wind was knocked out of me. I was in shock and felt dread and *fear*. What did this mean for my baby? My family? The next few days I experienced confusion, grief, and pain. But I also felt a fierce protectiveness over this little boy's life and body. This was still the same baby who grew inside me. I had to reconcile the boy I went to the hospital to welcome and the little baby boy in my arms with Down syndrome. My heart broke that I couldn't see past the diagnosis. A NICU nurse, and mom to a son with Ds, came and spoke with us the day after. Speaking to her was like sunlight shining through the clouds of my heart.

—ROSA TEXIDOR

My initial gut feeling was that I was carrying a baby girl with Down syndrome. [Since I was] twenty-nine, my OB only recommended the second trimester quad screen, and it came back "normal" with a risk of 1 in 7,000. I started preterm labor at twenty-five weeks. I was in and out of labor and delivery and had many non-stress tests and biophysical profiles. At thirty-six weeks, we were sent to a maternal-fetal medicine (MFM) specialist to investigate her kidneys further. At the MFM, her kidneys were perfect, but she had a complete atrioventricular canal heart defect. We were told of the potential of her having Down syndrome. Since I had been having preterm labor, the doctor advised against an amniocentesis. As soon as she was born, she was held up for me to see. I was able to spend an hour with her, breastfeeding and loving on her, before they took her to the NICU for her echocardiogram. Soon a doctor told us about their suspicions of Down syndrome. I remember saying "I know" and "Okay" and that was it. Even though I had a feeling about Ds and her heart pointed to Ds, it was still a shock and took many weeks to process.

—MARISA DUNN

Postnatal Diagnosis

Although a diagnosis of Down syndrome is usually made just after birth (assuming there has been no prenatal diagnosis), there are cases in which such a finding takes several weeks or months. All children are unique, and the physical characteristics of Down syndrome are not always present, but there may be signs as a child grows that a parent or medical professional will notice. While a late diagnosis is not common, some children are diagnosed further into their first year. If you have questions about your child not meeting milestones or having characteristics of Down syndrome, talk to your medical provider.

OUR EXPERIENCE: A Late Diagnosis

Strange though it may sound, discovering that my son had Down syndrome was like watching a flower bud unfurl. After an inexplicably anxious pregnancy and unsettled postpartum period, one day my son looked at me and *Down syndrome* skittered across my mind. My thoughts seemed so outlandish, I wondered if it was a psychotic break or postpartum depression. I searched online. What did “low-set ears” mean? All babies have flattened nose bridges. If I smooshed his hand one way, he had the palmar crease. Another way, his hand looked like mine. *No, impossible. Yes, it is.* I went on for days, bewildered. I held my baby and tears fell on him. He was almost two months old.

Before any testing, I knew. My son had Down syndrome.

The short bus, adoption, prenatal testing, disability—so many things clanged together in my mind. Then, the devastating guilt. Could he sense my distress and feel unloved? I realized that I still had important choices to make. What is independence? Achievement? Ability? Worth?

We cannot always choose the paths of our lives, but we can choose how we walk them. I have to nurture the flower that has been revealed to me; I chose happiness.

—JISUN LEE, BLOGGING AT KIMCHILATKES.COM

Sharing the News

Each family reacts differently to hearing about the diagnosis and chooses to share the news in the way that suits them best. Some want to share with everyone right away so it is all out in the open. Others want to process it more privately and tell family and friends in time. Still others never make an “announcement” or share the news broadly.

OUR EXPERIENCE: How We Shared the News

We told our closest friends and family in person or on the phone. Then, before leaving the hospital we announced on Facebook his arrival and that he also had Ds. I wanted to let everyone know about his diagnosis to help avoid any uncomfortable conversations and to let people know we were completely comfortable talking openly about it. I also told them this was all new to us and we welcomed any info and/or guidance. We received so many encouraging words and wonderful stories from everyone. It was a nice start to this unexpected journey.

—KRISTY CORRIGAN

We shared the news on Facebook after we had phoned all of our close family and told them individually. I'd say it was maybe eighteen hours after birth. We needed to have it out there, because we were reeling in shock. The response was wonderful—our friends and family are awesome.

—CATHLEEN SMALL

We let everyone meet her, then told them. I wanted people to not judge her based on a label.

—MEAGAN LOEKEN

We just told our parents and siblings. We had an emergency c-section at thirty-two weeks so I asked a coworker to share the news at work since they were already meeting one morning to pray for us. I was very emotional at that time and didn't want to go to work (an elementary school full of caring ladies) or get e-mails from a million teachers asking me about him. As for extended family, friends, and neighbors, we just tell them as we talk to them. I didn't feel like we needed to make a big announcement about it, but I also don't want anyone to think we are trying to hide it.

In hindsight (and now that we're far past the shock of it), it may have been easier to mention it on Facebook.

—MELISSA MCMURRAY

I didn't want anyone other than my fiancé, sister, and parents to visit us in the hospital. I couldn't keep myself together long enough for visits. But once we got the 'official' diagnosis (it took four days for blood tests to come back), we began texting close friends to tell them the news. We were so overwhelmed with information and were so afraid of the questions we might not be able to answer so we wanted to avoid phone calls or in-person visits at all costs. Within the first two weeks, most of our closest friends and family members knew. On Hunter's three-month birthday I started a blog and posted his birth story. At that point we realized the overwhelming support we actually had and that we don't always have to have the answers right away.

—ALICE FLUHRER

OUR EXPERIENCE: Beyond a Birth Diagnosis

When Ellie was born I knew my life was forever changed. I felt it, not in my heart but in the pit of my stomach. It was a fear that I would not be the same person from that day forward. A fear that my life would be filled with doctor's appointments, therapies, and research. That my duties as mother to my two older boys would be sacrificed. I worried for how my marriage would suffer because of this new journey I was about to take. I loved this tiny being with my whole soul but I worried that fighting for her would take away a part of who I was.

Those feelings in the pit of my stomach have since faded. The fear has grown into hope, and now I feel it in my heart. I now have a full, grateful, bursting-with-joy heart and it's hard for me to even put into words. I would like to try and share with you how Ellie has changed me. She has changed me in ways I never could have imagined.

Things I think about and look at differently . . .

1. Stopping to smell the roses.
2. Human rights.
3. Nutrition.
4. Understanding work *life*.
5. The importance of connections and support.
6. Being different is awesome.

I hear my boys *educating* their friends about Down syndrome. I hear them being more accepting and loving because of their sister. Now if we are out and about and they see someone who is differently abled, they will wave and say hello. This to me is the biggest part of how Ellie has changed not only me but all of us. Our hearts are bigger because of her. I also see her changing the hearts of our friends and family.

Yes Ellie, you have sure *changed* mama. And I am so glad you have. You are the little gift my soul needed. Thank you for opening my eyes to some of the biggest lessons I will ever learn in this lifetime. I am eternally grateful that you are mine. I can't wait to see what else you can teach me.

—TIFFANY STAFFORD, BLOGGING AT OUR3LILBIRDS.BLOGSPOT.COM

Resources

Finding Online Support

- BabyCenter—Down Syndrome Board: *http://community.babycenter.com/groups/a315/down_syndrome*
- Down Syndrome Diagnosis Network (DSDN): *www.dsdiagnosisnetwork.org*

- International Down Syndrome Coalition (IDSC): *http://theidsc.org/resources/support-for-parents.html*

Finding Local Support

- Down Syndrome Affiliates in Action: *www.dsaia.org/programs/find.html*
- Global Down Syndrome Foundation: *www.globaldownsyndrome.org/about-down-syndrome/resources/local-organizations*
- National Down Syndrome Congress: *www.ndsccenter.org/affiliate-directory*
- National Down Syndrome Society: *www.ndss.org/Resources/Local-Support*

Finding Information

- National Center for Prenatal and Postnatal Down Syndrome Resources: *http://downsyndromediagnosis.org*

Suggested Reading

- Becker, Amy Julia. *A Good and Perfect Gift: Faith, Expectations, and a Little Girl Named Penny*. Ada, MI: Bethany House, 2011.
- Hampton, Kelle. *Bloom: Finding Beauty in the Unexpected.* New York: William Morrow, 2013.
- Jacob, Jennifer. *Unexpected: Stories of a Down Syndrome Diagnosis*. Lulu.com, 2014.

- Soper, K. *Gifts: Mothers Reflect on How Children with Down Syndrome Enrich Their Lives*. Bethesda, MD: Woodbine House, 2007.

Part Two
THE JOURNEY

Chapter Four
Newborn to Six Months

Congratulations on your new baby!

Whether you had a prenatal or postnatal diagnosis of Down syndrome, the day of delivery and shortly thereafter can be a very challenging time emotionally and physically for you and your loved ones. A new member has joined your family and may have surprised you in more ways than one. Right away, lots of time is focused on the physical health of the child and establishing the right care plan. The first days can be a time of sadness and confusion for your family or a great celebration knowing the child has safely entered the world. Communication with medical professionals is key during the early months as you work to best meet and understand your child's needs. While there may be lots of anxiety in those first days, medical advances in recent decades have made a powerful difference for those with Down syndrome. The research and resources available to your family will allow you to get your child off to a wonderful start!

Dear New Parent,

Grasp your baby's finger. Snuggle your baby closely. Look into his or her eyes. Soak in all the new baby smells and sounds. The newborn time passes too quickly. Before you know it, your child will be running in all directions. Take this time to get to know your offspring and learn. Yes, your child has "designer genes" and is rockin' an extra chromosome. But before all that, she is *your* child. Give yourself grace and patience as you move forward together. You are going to rock this!

OUR EXPERIENCE: The First Moments

She came out fast and furious at eight pounds ten ounces and twenty-one inches long. The neonatologist came to see her and then whispered to me that her heart and lungs were great, but that she had Down syndrome. I thanked him, smiled, and told him that I knew she did. I cried tears of happiness as they put her on me for skin-to-skin and as I proclaimed to my husband how beautiful she was.

—JANESSA GROSS

When my son, Elijah, was born and we learned a few days later that he had Ds, I broke down. I was angry at the world. I questioned what I did to deserve a child with Ds.

—JASON MASONY

When he was plopped up on my chest, my first thought was "Oh, my God, he has Down syndrome." I repeatedly asked the doctor and nurses if he was "okay/fine/healthy" because I was too afraid to ask if he had Ds, but really I wanted to scream, "He has Down syndrome!" No one at the hospital said anything until thirty-two hours after birth (I hadn't even brought up my suspicions with my husband), and when they told us, I cried, held Gabe, and told him I loved him on repeat about 1,000 times.

—KRISTIE MAGNUSON

My emotions were everywhere . . . Trembling in fear I thought: Wait, what did [the doctor] just say? Is this really happening? I'm so scared to see her. My heart hurts. Will I ever be happy again? I love her; she's beautiful. I was chosen for her but what if I fail her? Lord, help me understand.

—KAY BROWN

Those First Days

First, and most important, *be kind to yourself.* You'll be subject to a lot of thoughts and emotions. There are no right or wrong feelings, just *your* feelings. You may have thoughts that surprise you and you wish you could take back. You may feel just fine about everything and not think twice about Down syndrome.

Take one day at a time and give yourself grace in those moments when a word, look, or touch seems to catch you off-guard and send you into a spiral of thoughts. Seek out the information you need, but try not to be consumed by online searches. Looking for stories of how other families, like yours, heard about the diagnosis? Read *Unexpected* by Jennifer Jacob at *www.missiont21.com* with free, downloadable stories of diagnoses.

OUR EXPERIENCE: The First Days

We came home after forty-eight hours even though Sulli was a twin and born at thirty-six weeks. She was totally big and healthy.

—PAIGE BRADLEY

Gracie was born with a complete patent ductus arteriosus (PDA) and atrioventricular canal defect (AV) canal defect, and we were all home together within three days of her birth. The only additional time she spent in the hospital was when she had her heart surgery at four and a half months old.

—JAMIE BRADFORD

The first few days can be summed up with one word: overwhelming. The shock of a birth diagnosis, paired with fear of the unknown, overshadowed the joy of our new baby. Thankfully we quickly emerged from the overwhelming fog and embraced our perfect little man. The constant worry didn't leave, but our team of doctors explained things so well and didn't add unnecessary stress. They quickly made us realize Zak was going to be fine and that he, in fact, was very healthy.

—BECKY BRATELY

Ben didn't have any extra time at the hospital-but he did have to be treated for jaundice for a little while. He was in the nursery under the lights and I was able to go feed him and visit him.

—DEBORAH TOMEI

We came home fourteen hours after birth with a complete atrioventricular septal defect and singular deformed valve. This was the first of my three children who I heard cry, that was pink and that I got to cut the cord. He was also the first who didn't end up in the special care nursery.

—JOHN WILKINSON-WITTS

Within two days, we were released to go home. Unfortunately on day seven we were readmitted so he could be under the lights for jaundice. He spent five more days there before we could bring him home.

—CHARI SASSIN

Isaiah had a seizure upon birth. Causes were unknown, but possibilities included a brain virus, blood on the brain, or perhaps something else. The situation was dire. Isaiah was being rushed to a NICU at a nearby specialty children's hospital. Expect months, at best, in the NICU, we were told. Isaiah spent a mere seven days in the NICU. Every test he had failed or had created major cause for concern at our birth hospital miraculously came back negative at the NICU, and through God's grace we were able to come home as a family.

—MICHELLE TESORI

Neonatal Intensive Care Unit Time

As you can see from the preceding stories, just because your baby is born with Down syndrome does not necessarily mean he'll need time in intensive care. However, a number of potential complications can arise with babies, whether born with Ds or not, and your child may need the support of a special care unit or neonatal intensive care unit (NICU) at the hospital. Common areas of concern for babies with Down syndrome include issues related to a premature birth, body temperature regulation, and maintaining oxygen levels. Even though not all babies with Ds spend time in the NICU, most will be evaluated by a NICU team, if one is available.

Care Team

Your baby may need to spend hours, days, weeks, or more in the care of the neonatology team. A neonatologist, a physician who specializes in the care of infants needing extra support, will be your child's primary-care provider during his or her stay in the NCIU. She will coordinate with other specialists to manage your child's care. A pediatric cardiologist, for example, will review your baby's heart echocardiogram, which provides details about the structures and functions of the heart. A pulmonologist and/or respiratory therapist may work to monitor your child's breathing needs. These specialists, along with others and the nursing staff, will be key points of contact and information during a NICU stay. Maureen Wallace, veteran NICU parent, offers this advice: "Spending time in the NICU is like going to Baby College. You are surrounded by experts, so ask questions and take notes." Read more tips from Maureen at *www.allparenting.com/my-family/articles/966161/advice-for-navigating-the-nicu*.

The Roller Coaster

Time in the hospital can be isolating and frustrating; many call it a roller-coaster ride. The emotions of a new diagnosis, paired with postpartum hormones, can make for a challenging time. There are few words to describe the moment you, as a patient, are discharged and leave the hospital without your baby. You may spend hours by a bedside waiting for a chance to snuggle your baby. You may pump round the clock to provide the "liquid gold" breastmilk for a tube feeding or bottle. You may have to travel hours from your hometown to the high-level NICU or stay nearby away from home. If you have other children, you may feel the pains of how to split your time. There will be good days and hard days, celebrations and struggles. Keep focused on your child and preparing for the day he or she will join you at home.

The March of Dimes suggests some ways for parents to cope with this period:

- Give yourself permission to cry and feel overwhelmed
- Establish a routine
- Connect with other NICU parents
- Explore your spiritual side
- Keep a journal
- Vent your frustration
- Celebrate when you can

- Accept the support of others
- Accept that you and your partner will react differently

Source: March of Dimes *(www.marchofdimes.org/baby/becoming-a-parent-in-the-nicu.aspx)*

The Balancing Act

Time in the NICU is also a balancing act for families. You or your partner (or both) may need to return to work. You may also need to share time between the hospital and other children at home. This can be a stress on your family, and it is important to communicate how everyone is coping during this time. As the March of Dimes suggests, you and your spouse may handle this experience very differently. A mother, for example, can provide breastmilk and be scheduled around the clock for pumpings and feedings, just as with any other newborn; dad may feel more directly removed in his NICU parenting role, but he can be the primary link to the older children, who need to understand what is going on. It is important that the two of you communicate.

NOTE FROM THE AUTHOR: THE WORLD OF NICU

The NICU really is its own little world. Parents who have done time in the NICU are a great resource for new parents to understand and explain things along the way. When our first child was born at thirty-two weeks, we were fortunate to have good friends who had had twins in the NICU a year earlier. Why did that help? The NICU has its own language and flow with which the general public is unfamiliar. Having someone to answer questions and vent frustrations to makes the experience a bit easier.

Once we knew more about the inner workings of the NICU, I was better able to be a team player as my daughter's mom. For me, the best part of that time was the hands-on parenting. I learned so much as a first-time mom-from the nurses, especially. Waiting for shift changes to hear updates, talking with the doctors at rounds, reading my child's medical records/charts: these were all ways that I could best advocate for my child. It was sometimes hard to speak up and ask questions, but I quickly realized that was my job. I was her mom now, and she needed me. I also tried to rest when I could. I knew I needed to be ready and rested for when she would finally be able to join us at home. Thirty days after she was born, we were able to go home together as a family.

—Jen

OUR EXPERIENCE: The Neonatal Intensive Care Unit (NICU)

My water broke at twenty-eight weeks. Those first forty-eight hours were some of the scariest moments of my life. The neonatologist came to talk to me about what I could expect when my son was born. I held out to thirty-one weeks. We were told to expect Camden to stay in the NICU for four to five weeks to grow and to learn to eat. It seemed so unnatural to leave the hospital without my son in my arms. I went to the hospital each day for almost nine weeks.

He was breathing on his own from the start. He had an IV for fluids and nutrition, and a tube from his mouth to his stomach for milk. He only needed time. I cried every single time I left him. I wanted him home. After four weeks, we tried to feed him with a bottle. This was by far his biggest obstacle. I started to lose hope; he just couldn't get it. I was dealing with the emotions from the diagnosis and from the NICU stay, and I was a wreck. I'm thankful for the amazing nurses [who were] patient and loving with him and comforting to me. It took him almost five more weeks, but he got to come home. Our family was finally complete.

—DIANE HILL

Bonding with Baby

Lots of emotions come with having a new baby. Some parents feel a struggle to bond and connect with their new baby with Down syndrome as they process the diagnosis. You might struggle to feel a connection if your baby has complex medical issues. When your child is in the NICU, for example, it may not be possible to hold and snuggle him immediately. Sometimes breastfeeding may not be successful, and you can't form the connection that brings. It is important to talk about this with your medical team and find ways of bonding. A great way to connect is through kangaroo holding (see the following section). This method of skin-to-skin contact can be a powerful way for you to connect with your new child. It may also help to seek out a counselor or therapist to talk with. Remember, be kind to yourself and use your family and friends for support.

Kangaroo Care

Kangaroo care, also called skin-to-skin, is a wonderful way to be close to your baby. It means holding your diapered baby on your bare chest (if you're the father) or between your breasts (if you're the mother). Be sure to put a blanket over your baby's back to keep him warm. If you are in the NICU, this may be limited depending on your baby's health. Let your baby's care team know you are interested in trying it out. Kangaroo care is a great way to connect and bond for parents and baby.

The benefits for your baby include the following:

- Regulates body temperature
- Regulates heart and breathing rates
- Helps baby gain weight
- Allows for increased amounts of deeper sleep
- Allows baby to spend more quiet awake time (rather than crying)
- Encourages breastfeeding

Kangaroo care also has benefits for you:

- Increases breastmilk production
- Decreases stress
- Encourages bonding and connection

Source: March of Dimes (*www.marchofdimes.org/baby/kangaroo-care.aspx*)

OUR EXPERIENCE: Bonding

I was terrified of breastfeeding. My OB said babies with Down syndrome don't feed well. I've always breastfed, and I've never been able to pump. This has been one of the biggest fears of this pregnancy for me. It was a bonding with my others and I already feel nervous about her and our bond.

—EMILY NEILSEN

I felt like I was forced into a room I really did not want to enter and was locked in . . . for the rest of my life. My son won't have Ds for six weeks, six months, or six years. Nothing will ever be the same again, and I wanted out. I think it all boiled down to change. I was so in love with my beautiful boy, but devastated to accept we were going to have to deal with Ds and all the negative stereotypes I had been exposed to in nursing school and in life. I felt so guilty. I later realized I had to peel back a part of myself I really didn't like to allow myself to truly express love to my son. He has changed me in the most beautiful way. I later asked my husband if he thought Jacob could sense my struggle. I needed to know that he felt his mommy loved him . . . He reassured me this was something I was dealing with on the inside and did not affect Jacob. Bonding is so tough because you are struggling to accept these changes when you really have absolutely *no* idea what it all means.

—KRISTY CORRIGAN

The Role of Medical Professionals

In the days immediately after your child's birth, evaluations and exams will be completed to best understand your new baby's well-being and specific medical needs. Today, much more is known about conditions such as heart defects that are commonly connected to Down syndrome. The good news is that these exams allow for treatment and support right away.

Many medical professionals and staff will visit your baby in the first days after he is born, and while it may seem overwhelming, it is necessary to make care decisions for the child. If a baby has or is suspected of having Down syndrome, the American Academy of Pediatrics (AAP) explains that a thorough physical examination of the baby should occur in the first twenty-four hours. The doctor will look for physical indicators for Ds and talk with families about Down syndrome. A pediatrician should also be available to talk with you and answer questions that you may have about Ds. Reach out to the medical team for support and guidance and ask questions as needed. You are your child's best advocate and you should be a part of the decision-making process.

During these first days, a hospital social worker may visit to talk about early intervention and other parent/child support programs provided by the state. The medical team should also provide a list of local resources and/or contacts for you to have on hand. You may or may not be ready to reach out right away, but having the information for when the time is right is key. In some areas, you may receive a welcome basket and information from a local Down syndrome organization.

NOTE FROM THE AUTHOR

In the first weeks, there may be a few things that seem unusual about your baby with Down syndrome, especially if you have had other children. Owen was our fourth child, and I noticed a few unusual things. After talking with lots of other parents and medical providers, I realized some of these nuances came with Down syndrome. It was nice to know these were things I could expect and when to look more closely. While they are not necessarily worrisome, you may notice the following things:

- **Hypotonia.** Hypotonia, or low tone, is a common feature of those with Down syndrome. Some doctors may describe your child as "floppy" or "lacking stability." In any case, you will probably notice your baby is extra snuggly. It may feel as if your infant has melted right into you as you hold her. Low tone means that your baby may take a little longer to meet milestones such as holding her head up or sitting. You also may notice your little one is extra flexible, another mark of hypotonia. Your therapists will help provide exercises to build up core strength over the years, and your baby will surely make progress. Until then, enjoy those extra sweet snuggles.

- **Sleep.** Your baby may sleep *a lot*. Of course, newborns always sleep quite a bit, but it surely will seem strange to see your child sleeping twenty hours a day. Babies with Down syndrome often sleep through the night after just a few weeks. I even recall my friend, who also had a newborn at the same time, asking what my "secret" was to getting a full night's sleep. I jokingly answered, "Down syndrome!" It is true. Babies with Down syndrome can be exceptionally sleepy to begin with, which can sometimes interfere with eating and weight gain. Sometimes, this extra sleep can be associated with heart conditions, but not always. If you are concerned, be sure to talk with your medical team, but know that extra sleep is very common in babies with Ds. Enjoy your own chance for rest while you can!
- **Congestion.** Does your baby sound as if his nose is always stuffy? This is also not uncommon in babies with Down syndrome. Because of those generally smaller-than-normal nasal passages, babies with Down syndrome tend to sound more congested than typical babies. If the baby is not uncomfortable, this is not a problem and there is no need to try and clear the congestion. If the congestion is causing discomfort, humidifiers, bulb syringes, and saline solution may help alleviate some of this-be sure to use them gently and sparingly. The NoseFrida Snotsucker is another tool that some parents rely on. It is a parent-powered nasal aspirator and it really does the job! For

more details, visit *www.nosefrida.com*. Whatever tools you choose to use may not completely resolve the congestion, but this is not something to worry about if your baby is happy, eating well, and not uncomfortable. Often, it just takes time for baby's nasal passages to grow. Families report a big difference with the levels of congestion between the six- and nine-month marks. While congestion is bothersome, it's not necessarily harmful. If you are ever worried about baby's breathing, be sure to contact your medical team.

- **Goopy Eyes.** Along with those smaller nasal passages, your baby may have narrow nasolacrimal ducts (the tubes that connect the eye with the back of the nose). These tubes are typically very curvy and narrow and can become clogged. A narrow duct is more likely to become blocked and cause the eyes to water more frequently, putting the child at slightly greater risk for infection. If your child has discharge and crusty eyes, try to wipe her face with a cold washcloth. Some nursing mothers also believe in using small amounts of breastmilk to massage in the corner of the baby's eye. An eye or sinus infection is also possible and usually easily treated with antibiotics, so be sure to discuss this with your medical team if you find swollen or matted-shut eyes.

—Jen

Managing Health Care

In addition to finding the right medical team, it is also important to learn about things you may experience with your child with Down syndrome. There are great resources and professionals available to help you navigate your child's care.

It is important for you to have a good understanding of what the American Academy of Pediatrics Guidelines recommend for children with Down syndrome. Part of this means establishing a team of medical professionals to ensure your child's health care is well managed. Some parents are frustrated to discover their physicians are inexperienced in caring for a patient with trisomy 21. However, just because your chosen medical professional is not well versed in all the care aspects of a new child with Down syndrome, this does not mean that she cannot be an effective partner for you. Some parents have found that a physician's willingness to learn, listen, and collaborate are her most important qualities.

Depending on location, you may have access to a Down syndrome clinic or a developmental pediatrician (see *www.ndss.org/Resources/Health-Care/Health-Care-Providers*). Along with a primary-care provider overseeing your child's care, the Ds clinic generally includes a team of professionals who evaluate and provide recommendations for therapy, treatments, and resources. You may also seek access to a developmental pediatrician, another partner to work with as you manage your child's needs.

The first months of life with a child with Down syndrome can be some of the most challenging, as far as medical appointments go. Medical professionals recommend visits with several specialists during your baby's first six months. An advantage to meeting with these professionals in determining what additional needs your child may have is that you are building a network of professionals to whom you will have access as your child grows. These appointments also allow you to have a greater understanding and awareness for potential risks in the future. Sometimes a medical team will recommend seeing all or most of these specialists in the first few weeks; at other times your primary care provider may organize the key tests and you may only need to see the specialists recommended by your primary care provider or developmental specialist based on the specific needs of your baby.

Medical professionals who may be a part of your team include:

- Cardiologist (to evaluate for, monitor, and treat any heart defects)
- Ophthalmologist (to evaluate vision/eyes)
- Ear, Nose, and Throat specialist (to manage ears, nose, and throat concerns, including tonsils, adenoids, and ear tubes)
- Audiologist (to address hearing concerns)
- Gastro-intestinal specialist (to monitor the baby's digestive system)
- Endocrinologist (to check on thyroid, growth)
- Pulmonologist (to monitor lung/breathing concerns, including pulmonary hypertension and apnea)

What to Ask a Medical Professional

1. Does he have experience with treating other patients with a diagnosis that can impact development?
2. Does her health-care philosophy match yours?
3. Is this someone with whom you can communicate effectively?
4. Will this physician connect you with the resources you may need?

According to the American Academy of Pediatrics, Questions to Ask When Interviewing a Physician Include:

- What medical school did the pediatrician attend, and where did he or she undergo postgraduate and residency training?
- What is the doctor's policy on taking and returning phone calls? Is there a nurse in the office who can answer routine questions?
- Does the doctor communicate clearly, using layman's language (not medical jargon) to explain illnesses and treatments, and does the doctor make an effort to ensure that all your questions are answered?
- How are visits for acute illnesses handled? Can you make an appointment on short notice if your child needs to see the pediatrician because of a sore throat or an infection, for example?

Having the right medical team in place allows your child to receive the best care and for you to have excellent resources and information available over the years. This powerful partnership will also better equip you, as a parent, to best advocate for your child and provide for her current and future needs. If possible, contact your local Down syndrome organization or mentor families in the area for references and information on the medical professionals they have experience with.

AAP Care Guidelines

The American Academy of Pediatrics (AAP) provides helpful guidelines for parents and providers to monitor your baby's wellness over the years. It includes areas that could be potential areas of concern. These guidelines are intended to be reviewed at well-child appointments. As a parent, you may find it helpful to print the guidelines out and have them with you to refer to and share with the doctor. Many doctors will find this helpful and be glad to have the guidelines on hand during your visit: *www.healthychildren.org/English/health-issues/conditions/developmental-disabilities/Documents/Health_Care_Information_for_Families_of_Children_with_Down_Syndrome.pdf*.

Growth Charts

It is important to monitor your child's growth, especially over the first years. In the past, physicians have referred to growth charts specifically for babies and children with Down syndrome. In 2011, the AAP changed the recommendation to follow children with Down syndrome on the typical charts. This is due, in part, to the outdated information that no longer applies with the standard of care children receive today. Some physicians may still use the Ds charts and some provide the option to view your child's growth on both. If your baby was born prematurely, the Ds chart may be a tool to consider as it includes data for lower weights. Regardless of what you and your medical team choose, it is important to monitor your child's progress to ensure he is following his growth curve.

Health-Care Notebooks

A care notebook can become an important tool for your family and medical professionals. Electronic medical records are not yet able to organize and communicate information across institutions and across many years of care. Keeping a concise record of past care helps keep your care team organized and focused on the specific needs of your child. The Swindells Center, located in Oregon, defines it as a personal health record that helps parents coordinate the complex records of their child's care, services, and providers. It becomes a running record of medical care, treatment, concerns, and needs, a specific place for you to record all that is going on and to access this information quickly if the need arises. For more details on creating your own care notebook, visit *www.321mama.com/2014/12/care-notebooks-worth-effort.html.*

OUR EXPERIENCE: Care Notebooks

When our son was born, a friend suggested I start a care notebook for him. I was skeptical if I'd ever really use it, especially since his medical needs were pretty typical at the time. But I went ahead and downloaded some forms online, put them into a binder, and added some basic binder accessories. I filled it out and dutifully carried it to our first few doctor appointments. To my surprise, it was more useful than I imagined, especially since we've added a lot of "-ologists" to our team of medical care providers. Now, two years later, I keep it updated and take it to every appointment. Someone always has a question about when we last saw Dr. ABC, or when our next visit would be with Dr. XYZ. Or how much he weighed at every appointment for the past year (yes, I really got that question!). I don't have to remember details as long as I have my notebook with me. Plus, our doctors get to see super-cute pictures of our son, which has opened up some great conversations, and, I think, helps them to see him as a person, not just a patient."

—HEATHER HICKS, BLOGGING AT *WWW.321MAMA.COM*

DS-Connect

If you don't want to maintain a care notebook, you can use DS-Connect: The Down Syndrome Registry. This system is run by the National Institutes of Health, which created it to encourage research in the area of Down syndrome so that health-care professionals and scientists can better understand how to help those with Ds. After you register your child with DS-Connect, you can use the registry as a means of record keeping. Site members also have access to generalized data from the registry, including occurrences for medical conditions. For more information, visit *https://dsconnect.nih.gov*.

Baby's First Checkups

The AAP recommends that physicians should also complete a thorough checkup shortly after your baby with Ds is born. Your physician and/or specialists will look most closely at your baby's:

- Heart
- Feedings
- Eyes
- Hearing
- Digestion
- Breathing
- Bloodwork

Regardless of whether your OB performed a fetal echocardiogram if there was a prenatal diagnosis of Ds, a pediatric cardiologist should administer another one after birth. It is a quick, noninvasive test that looks like an ultrasound done over the baby's chest. Because up to 50 percent of those with Down syndrome have at least one heart defect, this test will allow doctors to best manage your child's cardiac care. Your doctor may refer you to a pediatric cardiologist to perform the test. Generally, a heart defect will be evaluated and monitored as the baby grows. Some defects will require surgery, while others will correct on their own in time. Some repairs may need to happen soon. Other surgeries require babies to be a little larger and stronger and may not happen until the child is closer to six months old. With proper medical care and experienced surgeons, the success rate for repairs has never been higher. Visit Chapter 5 for more details on heart surgery.

COMMON HEART DEFECTS			
Defect	**Abbreviation**	**Issue**	**Treatment**
Atrioventricular Canal Defect	Complete AV Canal	A single hole in the wall between both the upper two chambers and the lower two chambers	Surgically closed
Ventricular Septal Defect	VSD	Hole in the wall between the lower two chambers	Surgically closed
Atrial Septal Defect	ASD	Hole in the wall between the two upper chambers	Surgically closed
Patent Ductus Arteriosus	PDA	Connection remains open between the pulmonary artery and aorta	Will likely resolve on its own
Patent Foramen Ovale	PFO	Flap does not seal after birth between the upper right and left chambers	Often closes on its own—sometimes surgically closed
Tetralogy of Fallot	ToF	A complex defect with a hole in the wall between the lower two chambers; the pulmonary artery is narrow, increasing the pressure needed for the right heart to pump blood to the lungs; the aorta is shifted towards the right; all of this together causes some blood to bypass the lungs and pass into the aorta unoxygenated.	Surgically repaired (by age 3–6 months)

Source: Boston Children's Hospital: *www.childrenshospital.org*

View a text version of this table

OUR EXPERIENCE: Heart Defects

On the fetal echo they saw an *atrial septal defect* (ASD) and moderate ventricular septal defect (VSD). When they repeated the echocardiogram at birth, the VSD had decreased in size. At the follow-up, three months later, it had closed. We continue to monitor the ASD and it has decreased too and is now classified as a PFO. No surgery will be needed!

—CRISTINA ROTHFUSS

I was told my daughter was 100 percent healthy. There were no heart defects [apparent] after two echocardiograms during pregnancy. I also had a sonogram monthly because of my age. The day after she was born, they suspected she had Down syndrome so they did another echocardiogram. We found out she had a complete AV canal defect. She had open-heart surgery (OHS) when she was a few months old. Now, a year after, she is doing great!

—DAWN BELLEROSE

We found her heart defect at birth as they suspected Ds and did an echo to check her over. Everyone figured it would be fine since no one could hear anything. A few days later, they told us she had a VSD. She was just about six and a half months at surgery. Leading up to the surgery was the scary part, and every appointment we wondered if it was going to be the day they decide it is time to operate. I was relieved when it finally was time. The day of surgery, I was much calmer than I thought I would be. I was sure I would cry when I had to hand her over. The time went really fast. The first night was the hardest, not being able to hold her and watching her cry. The silent cry was the worst. We left four days later and it was over. She recovered very quickly.

—SIERRA TRAN

Ryan was thirteen weeks old when we handed him over for heart repair. I leaned on my faith and family for strength . . . and Google. I found Cora Bean's blog with helpful hints for the actual surgery and hospital stay. I honestly think there isn't any way to really prepare; it was the hardest day of my life. We spent five days in the pediatric ICU and never looked back!

—MANDY RAMZAN

Feedings

Depending on other conditions, such as heart defects and hypotonia, feeding may be a challenge. Babies with Down syndrome can be sleepier than typical children, which can cause them to fall asleep while eating. Although babies may get off to a slow start, most are able to successfully breastfeed or bottle-feed. If you're breastfeeding, the support of an experienced lactation consultant may provide the guidance you need to successfully nurse a baby with low tone or who is extra sleepy. If your child is slow to gain weight, chokes on feeds, or develops respiratory concerns, your doctor may refer you for a swallow study to gain more information. Feeding tubes, like a nasogastric (NG tube) or gastrostomy (G-tube), may be necessary for a small percentage of babies to receive proper nutrition.

OUR EXPERIENCE: Breastfeeding

I was determined to breastfeed. We struggled with her being very sleepy and a weak latch at first. On the third day of her barely taking anything, a nurse told us that I could pump. She showed us how we could finger-feed her with a syringe. This was our go-to method of feeding the first couple weeks but she was still not gaining weight well by week three. My husband finally convinced me at that time that we should start her on supplemental formula. (I was initially against it.) But once we started breastfeeding and supplementing some formula afterward, she started gaining strength. I wish I hadn't waited so long to really start supplementing. We used formula as needed until she was about four months. Then I was gradually able to work her back to full-time breastfeeding. A supportive family and husband helped the most. I shouldn't have waited so long to start pumping in the hospital and pumped for all her missed feedings. I didn't realize that I should be pumping and syringe-/bottle-feeding her what she wasn't strong enough to get for herself. Thus my milk supply dropped, and so did her strength. She breastfed until she was one year!

—SHERI SELPH

Advice from a Lactation Consultant

International Board Certified lactation consultant Sarah Rush Stevens says, "The most important investment a new mother can make in her breastfeeding success is to start expressing milk as soon as possible—ideally within six hours of birth. The body decides how much milk to make over the long term based on how much is removed in the first few days of the baby's life. Babies with Down syndrome may not remove much milk at first, even if they are spending a lot of time at the breast. So removing milk, with pumping or with hand expression, helps to make sure there's enough milk available when the baby is ready to take all feeds at the breast. Hospitals have pumps available in the mother-baby and NICU areas, but nurses often forget to offer them. There is so much activity in the first few hours after the baby is born, especially when there are big health concerns, that the pump may be low priority for health-care providers. It can help for the new mother to designate someone else, such as a partner, friend, or other support person, to follow up on her pump request so that she is free to take in information about the status of her baby."

Most babies with Ds can breastfeed, although it may take a bit longer to establish and depends upon the baby's medical needs. There are great resources, such as a hospital lactation consultant, to help support mothers who nurse. Also check out *http://kellymom.com/ages/newborn/nb-challenges/down-syndrome* for helpful tips and resources.

OUR EXPERIENCE: Breastfeeding

Our experience was relatively easy. We had to use a nipple shield for the first six to eight weeks, but once he latched without it, we were good to go until thirteen months. At that time, he started teething and basically unexpectedly weaned himself. I'm still pumping, but I haven't had any luck getting him to latch. I wanted to breastfeed as long as possible, but I'm so thankful I was able to go over a year!

—NATALIE PALIN

The doctors warned that because of her heart (atrioventricular canal defect) she may not have the stamina to keep it up and do it long term. A lactation consultant came to visit me, but [the baby] had a great latch and started gaining weight so we never needed her services. However, I often say Britton never got the memo that her heart didn't work; she never really went into heart failure and gained seven pounds in the five months between her birth and surgery. She did great from the beginning!

—STACEY VANDERBENT

Ivan was six weeks early, so they told me his "sucking reflex" hadn't developed yet and that it was going to take time to teach him. Per the doctor and lactation nurse, I breastfed every two hours and pumped every other hour . . . for two days! I was a crying, exhausted, emotional mess. I topped him off with a finger tube and expressed milk. The third day he got it, and we haven't looked back since.

—NADIA PAPAGNI

Our breastfeeding journey began with doctors saying it wasn't possible to exclusively breastfeed a baby with both Down syndrome and an AV canal defect. Amidst feeling out of control we received two blessings: a lactation consultant who believed in us, and a wonderful cardiologist. Bonnie was not able to take a bottle, so supplementation to assist with weight gain was not an option. Our lactation consultant, Sarah, worked with us throughout our journey. She provided both the support and community we desperately needed. If you're in a similar situation, find a Sarah. Find someone apart from family to cheer you on when everyone says it's impossible. It's not impossible. Lastly, despite our pediatrician's concern about Bonnie's slow weight gain, we had a cardiologist who felt she was on track. While I spent nights wishing Bonnie was on the growth charts, that wasn't her story. We chose to trust our cardiologist. After Bonnie's AV canal repair, she took off. Anxiety disappeared from our weekly weight checks and she began exceeding her weight goals. Bonnie is an exclusively breastfed baby. We started feeling alone and ended with a community that believes in our breastfeeding journey. I am forever grateful.

—CRYSTAL TILLMAN

Eyes

Newborn eyes should be evaluated for cataracts and blocked tear ducts. After birth, a physician will look for a red reflex to determine whether your baby has cataracts. If cataracts are suspected, you should arrange for them to be promptly evaluated and treated by a pediatric opthalmologist. Blocked tear ducts (dacryostenosis) generally occur in babies with trisomy 21 because the eye ducts tend to be smaller. Often massage and topical treatments will help. If this persists as your child grows, an opthalmologist might need to surgically open the ducts.

How to Help Blocked Tear Ducts

Many infants with Down syndrome have issues with a goopy, crusty eye or two. Those narrow tear ducts are the cause. While it is not necessarily harmful to the baby, it can cause discomfort. Use a warm washcloth to gently wipe across the closed eyelid several times a day. Gently massage the inner corner of the eye; this can also help to reduce the drainage. If you are a nursing mother, consider using a bit of breastmilk to carefully massage your child's eye.

Hearing

Up to 60 percent of people with Down syndrome will experience a form of hearing loss at some point. A newborn hearing screen, brainstem auditory evoked response (BAER), or otoacoustic emission (OAE) test will be completed before you and your baby are sent home from the hospital. Depending on the results, you may need to follow up with an ENT specialist or audiologist and have an auditory brainstem response (ABR). During the ABR, doctors look for two types of hearing loss:

1. **Conductive.** Sound does not move well from the inner, middle, and outer ear and causes sounds to be muffled or faint. This can be caused by fluid, wax, and infection, among other things. This can be solved medically or surgically.
2. **Sensorineural.** There is damage to the inner ear or the nerve path from the inner ear to the brain. This is the most common form of permanent loss and can be caused by certain illnesses, head trauma, or malformation of the ear and causes sound to be unclear or muffled. This cannot be fixed medically or surgically.

It is important to determine how well the baby can hear because proper hearing allows for speech development. If there are hearing issues, speech delays are more common, so it is important that you and your doctor monitor your baby's hearing in the first months/years. For more information, visit *www.asha.org/public/hearing/Types-of-Hearing-Loss*.

As mentioned, babies with Down syndrome tend to have small ear canals. The tiny canals can cause wax buildup, and their shape can cause fluid to remain in the ear; both impact hearing. It is not uncommon for babies to fail hearing tests in the first months and then pass once the canals have grown a bit larger. It can be frustrating, but it is important to continue to monitor to determine what your baby's problem really is—small, fluid-filled ear canals or true hearing loss. For some babies, your doctor may insert tubes in her or his ears. Others will need hearing aids for temporary or permanent hearing support.

NOTE FROM THE AUTHOR

Owen did not pass one single hearing test until the day we went to pick up hearing aids. In the hospital they tested him several times, but due to fluid or tiny ear canals he never "passed" the screenings. At just a few months old, we took him for an ABR, and that showed minor hearing loss in one ear and moderate loss in the other. We waited a few more months and completed another ABR. Slightly better results, but still enough hearing loss for us to consider hearing aids. We also decided to place ear tubes to see if that would resolve the issue. Testing after the tubes remained the same. I knew how important speech development would be for Owen, and I did not want to take any chance that hearing would be a barrier for him. At nine months, we met with an audiologist and [he was] fitted for hearing aids. The day before his hearing aid placement, we visited the ENT who still saw no fluid, further convincing us that this was permanent hearing loss. The next day, the audiologist ran a few more hearing tests to best set the hearing aids. This time, he passed each one! We believe the larger issue was wax buildup in those tiny canals and [we] now visit the ENT regularly to have them cleaned out and checked for fluid. For more on testing, like the ABR, visit *www.asha.org/public/hearing/Hearing-Testing*.

—Jen

OUR EXPERIENCE: Treating Hearing Loss

Shortly after [his] birth, I was convinced my son was deaf. He did not stir as I tapped against the plastic. The next morning my fears subsided as he passed his newborn hearing screen with flying colors. At four months old, while sedated after open-heart surgery (OHS), the doctor recommended an ABR. Afterward, the audiologist explained the test showed moderate to severe conductive loss in his left ear and moderate loss in his right ear. She discussed the frequency he could hear at and at what decibel. He could hear sounds, but they were muffled—like being under water. Everett's eardrums showed very poor mobility most likely due to fluid. [The doctors] recommended hearing aids, and Everett was fitted for bone conduction hearing aids at seven months. His hearing loss also qualified him for intensive speech therapy as well as sign-language instruction. These services have been invaluable in his development of communication skills. Many states have programs for deaf and hard-of-hearing children that provide loaner hearing aids and communication instruction. Be vigilant about things that can affect your child's hearing, [such as] frequent ear infections [and] respiratory infections. Insist on hearing tests, and if a problem is noticed, make sure the follow-up is quick.

—AMBER SMITH

Digestion

Along with feedings, you should monitor digestion concerns and discuss them with your doctor, especially in the first days. It is important for your baby to have proper nutrition and to ensure her digestive system is properly functioning. Considerations for physicians examining infants with Ds include:

1. **Duodenal Atresia.** Often referred to as double bubble because of how it is visualized on an ultrasound, this is a condition when the small bowel does not properly develop. A space occurs in the intestine, and contents of the stomach cannot empty into the intestines. This condition can be found

before or after birth and is corrected with surgery within a few days. Symptoms generally present a day or two after birth and include:

- No stool passed
- Swollen belly from gas
- Vomiting; vomit may be yellow or greenish in color
- Lack of appetite

2. **Constipation.** This is very common in children with Down syndrome and is often managed through diet. Because of low tone, the digestive system can work more slowly, causing constipation. Talk with your doctor about management options.

Constipation

Poop is a necessary part of parenting, but it becomes an even greater challenge when there is too much or not enough. Because of low muscle tone, babies and children with Down syndrome tend to be constipated. You should speak with your child's doctor if issues arise. Blood in the stool is never normal, and you should contact your doctor right away. You might consider evaluating your baby's fluid/dietary intake and beginning a probiotic to help regulate the digestive system, especially if you notice infrequent or very hard stools. For chronic constipation, talk with your doctor about management options.

3. **Hirschsprung's disease.** This can be a factor for babies with Down syndrome. If a baby has not had a bowel movement in the first few days, your doctor may do an examination. Hirschsprung's is a condition that involves missing nerve cells in the muscles in the large intestine that prevent stool from passing through. Surgery is often necessary to resolve the issue. Symptoms in infants include:

    - Not having a bowel movement in the first forty-eight hours of life
    - Gradual marked swelling of the abdomen
    - Gradual onset of vomiting
    - Fever

4. **Gastroesophageal reflux disease (GERD).** This may be a concern for infants and children with Down syndrome. GERD occurs when stomach acid refluxes into and irritates the esophagus. Common symptoms are:

    - Frequent or recurrent vomiting
    - Frequent or persistent cough
    - Refusing to eat or difficulty eating (choking or gagging with feeding)
    - Crying with feeding or after feeding
    - Heartburn, gas, or abdominal pain

Breathing

Stridor (high-pitched) wheezing or noisy breathing are common in babies with Down syndrome, often due to those small or floppy airways. You may well notice some form of unusual breathing with your child, either immediately after she's born or later. If the matter is serious enough, your doctor may refer you to a pulmonologist, who specializes in the lungs. A sleep study may also be performed to determine a course of action and possible treatment. Some children will require additional oxygen for a portion of the day or night or full-time depending on needs. It's possible your child suffers from one of the following:

1. **Apnea.** Infants may be assessed for apnea (pauses in breathing while asleep) and oxygen desaturations (decreasing levels of oxygen in the blood) before leaving the hospital, which is especially important when low tone persists. Sometimes, babies are monitored using a car-seat safety evaluation before leaving the hospital. During this test, babies are placed into the infant car seat/carrier and their heart rate and breathing are measured. There are two forms of sleep apnea: obstructive and central. Obstructive sleep apnea is the most common and is caused by relaxed throat muscles. Central sleep apnea happens when the message to the muscles that control breathing are not properly received by the brain. A pulmonologist is the specialist that will work with you on apnea.
2. **Laryngomalacia.** Softening of the tissue in the voice box, laryngomalacia or "floppy airway," is another condition that is more common in infants with Down syndrome. In a 2012 study published by the *International Journal of Pediatrics*, laryngomalacia was found to be the most common cause of stridor (noisy airflow due to narrow airways) in newborns; a high percentage of those had Down syndrome. Your doctor will monitor for this condition but may also suggest you consult a pulmonologist. Symptoms associated with laryngomalacia include:

- Feeding difficulties
- Poor weight gain (failure to thrive)
- Regurgitation of food (vomiting or spitting up)

- Choking on food
- Gastroesophageal reflux (spitting up acid from the stomach)
- Chest and/or neck retractions (chest and/or neck sinking in with breathing)
- Cyanosis (turning blue)
- Apnea (pauses in breathing)

Inspiratory Stridor

Infants with laryngomalacia have intermittent noisy breathing when breathing in. This is called inspiratory stridor. The inspiratory stridor may be better or worse in different positions; it very often becomes worse with agitation, crying, excitement, feeding, or when your baby is positioned or sleeps on his back. These symptoms are often present at birth or occur within the first ten days of life. However, the noisy breathing of laryngomalacia may begin any time during the first year of life. Symptoms will often increase or get worse over the first few weeks after diagnosis. Most infants with laryngomalacia outgrow the noisy breathing by twelve to eighteen months.

Bloodwork

Starting after birth, doctors will take blood samples from your child often throughout childhood to measure and monitor several areas. Physicians will test your baby for:

1. **Hypothyroidism.** This occurs when the thyroid makes little or no thyroid hormone. Doctors monitor for abnormal levels

of T4 or TSH hormones. A pediatrician or endocrinologist (a specialist whose focus includes the thyroid) will coordinate this care. If left untreated, thyroid concerns may lead your baby to have decreased cognitive ability, so this is something to be taken very seriously. According to Boston Children's Hospital, treatment may include replacing deficient hormones. Some children will require hormone replacement therapy for the rest of their lives, while others appear to outgrow the disorder, often by the age of three. It is often asymptomatic, but some symptoms that should make you think of hypothyroidism include:

- Jaundice (yellowing of the skin, eyes, and mucous membranes)
- Hoarse cry
- Poor appetite
- Umbilical hernia (navel protrudes out)
- Constipation
- Slow bone growth

Source: *www.childrenshospital.org/conditions-and%20treatments/conditions/h/hypothyroidism/overview*

2. **Transient Myeloproliferative Disorder (TMD).** This is a form of leukemia that occurs in newborns with Ds. According to the American Association of Pediatricians, TMD is found almost exclusively in newborn infants with Down syndrome and is relatively common among them (10 percent). TMD usually regresses spontaneously within the first three months of life, but there is an increased risk (10–30 percent) of later onset of leukemia for these patients.

Source: *http://pediatrics.aappublications.org/content/128/2/393.full.pdf*

When to Worry

With all the tests doctors run on your baby in the first days and weeks, it's inevitable that you'll worry. Families report feeling as if they were waiting for the other shoe to drop each time a test was run. Any little thing may cause you anxiety. A great example of this is petechiae, a red, dotted rash that with one moment's Internet search can send you down a dark path of concern. In infants, petechiae can be a benign response to a virus, skin irritation, a fit of crying, or a sign of an underlying condition that needs attention. The only way to know is through a doctor's visit and bloodwork. Within a short time, you will have results and know how to move forward. It is important to know what to expect, but it is also essential to keep calm and take things day to day.

OUR EXPERIENCE: TMD

After many weeks of health scares for my unborn son, I was induced and he was born at thirty-five weeks. The pediatrician came in the next day with a concerned look on her face. The doctor found blasts in my baby's blood. I thought to myself, blasts? Blasts are cancer. What does this mean? We were immediately sent to a hematologist/oncologist. Even with my nursing degree, I felt my mind exploding.

Camden was born with TMD. Most doctors had never seen Camden's type of leukemia before. At two months of age Camden was extremely jaundiced. The doctors were worried that the neonatal leukemia was attacking his liver. His labs were all out of whack. His white blood cells were 80,000. Nothing was normal. We were put in the hospital to do a workup for a possible liver transplant, get a blood transfusion, and possibly get chemo. Camden got his blood transfusion, and the next morning all his labs had corrected themselves. Including his liver function. The doctors said it was idiopathic. Which is a big word for "we don't know what happened." A few weeks after that Camden's limbs swelled up really big and no one could tell us why. At six months the TMD resolved. We saw the hematologist/oncologist less and less.

—MEGHAN ROBERSON

Baby-Wearing and Ds

One of the decisions you'll make in the first weeks your baby is home is how to carry her. The use of infant carriers and baby slings is a common practice around the world. You may baby-wear for closeness and bonding or convenience to get a few things done with a sleeping baby who loves to be held. Many of the same benefits mentioned for kangaroo care (see the concepts discussed earlier in this chapter) apply to baby-wearing too. Even moms who are veterans of baby-wearing may wonder if this is the right thing to do with their new little one.

While some professionals recommend certain styles of carriers over others based on your child's physical needs, there are lots of carrier options and resources available. For example, if your child has loose hips, it may be better to choose a carrier that will bring her legs together rather than spread them apart. All babies with low tone need extra attention to head position when baby-wearing. For support, contact *http://babywearinginternational.org*.

OUR EXPERIENCE: Baby-wearing

When I was pregnant, avid baby-wearing mama that I am, I was busy dreaming and planning to wrap a newborn again. One of my first questions was, how am I going to need to adapt baby-wearing to meet our needs? Of course there is no way to predict or plan or know ahead of time which characteristics or challenges your baby might have, but on the whole, there isn't too much extra to worry about [regarding] wearing a baby with Down syndrome. The biggest challenge for us was hypotonia, the low muscle tone that makes Cop a little weaker and floppier than his brother was. This means you have to keep a better eye on positioning when wearing.

Some babies have open-heart surgery or need feeding tubes, and they can all benefit from baby-wearing. Baby-wearing fosters bonding and closeness, can make breastfeeding easier and more convenient, and can help you meet your own needs and the needs of the rest of the family. Baby-wearing can bring mobility and inclusion to kids whose physical developmental delays might otherwise slow them down, and of course wearing your baby will make it easier to get through all those appointments.

—DREA EISENBURG, BLOGGING AT *WWW.THEMAIDENMETALLURGIST.COM* AND CO-FOUNDER OF 321CARRY.ORG

Sibling Relationships

After learning about a diagnosis of Down syndrome, parents often wonder how having a special needs child will impact existing siblings and future children. In 2011, Brian Skotko, Susan Levine, and Richard Goldstein conducted a study involving more than 800 siblings of people with Down syndrome and found that "More than 96 percent of brothers/sisters that responded to the survey indicated that they had affection toward their sibling with Ds; and 94 percent of older siblings expressed feelings of pride. Less than 10 percent felt embarrassed, and less than 5 percent expressed a desire to trade their sibling in for another brother or sister without Ds. Among older siblings, 88 percent felt that they were better people because of their siblings with Ds, and more than 90 percent plan to remain involved in their sibling's lives as they become adults. The vast majority of brothers and sisters describe their relationship with their sibling with Ds as positive and enhancing." Find the full research article at *www.brianskotko.com*.

OUR EXPERIENCE: Siblings

The very first time I held Tessa in my arms, her doctor shared that she suspected my new baby might have Down syndrome. Shocked by this news, my husband and I fell apart as we tried to collect our emotions and our thoughts. We thought about Tessa's six-year-old brother, wondering how this unexpected twist would affect him and our family as a whole. But he loved her without hesitation because he knew no less, holding her and kissing her forehead so full of pride. The minute he met her, he looked at her the way I should have been since hearing the suspicion of Down syndrome—without apprehension or fear. From that moment forward what I wanted him—and everyone else—to feel was empowered by things unexpected.

We shared Tessa's diagnosis with her brother months after her birth, and he expressed even more pride and love for his little sister. As we watched Tessa grow into our family, we did not hesitate to expand our family further. Twenty months later, we welcomed another baby girl into our lives. The dynamic of our children's relationship is exactly how we imagined it would be. Choosing love over fear was by far the easiest and best choice we ever made.

—BECKY CAREY, AUTHOR OF *47 STRINGS: TESSA'S SPECIAL CODE*

Watching Piper and Jude together is [a] rare glimpse into a love story where love comes unconditionally. Piper's love for Jude was unwavering and unquestioning. The last time Piper was having an anxiety attack, Horacio was helping her to breathe through it. He told her to imagine something that made her feel better. Later she told me she imagined holding Jude's hand. The same thing occurred today when she was asked to share something she was grateful for. She hesitated, unsure of the word, so I whispered to her "What makes you happy?" "Jude," she said loudly, beaming at her sister.

We talked a couple of weeks ago about her anxiety, and she confessed to me that she worries about Jude dying. When Jude was in the hospital with *respiratory syncytial virus* (RSV), it really scared Piper to see her with tubes in her nose. For a moment, I floundered because I am scared for Jude too. Right now she's healthy, but I am all too aware this can change. So I told Piper what I tell myself: "We can't know the future for any of us. But we can love now without holding anything back. We need to bask in this moment. This love."

—GINGER STICKNEY, BLOGGING AT *WWW.GREENTEAGINGER.COM*

Get Connected

The Ds community is an (unexpectedly) wonderful place to be. Once indoctrinated into the "club," the amount of support you'll receive really is unbelievable. There are playdates, events, classes, conventions, meet-ups, online groups—many ways to learn about Down syndrome and connect with other families. Connect when you are interested and ready.

Local Groups

Just as you can turn to local groups when your child is first diagnosed with Ds, whether prenatal or postnatal, so too these groups can offer you support after your child is born and growing. Larger cities may have several Down syndrome organizations available as a resource for you. Whether you get in touch with an official city or state Down syndrome organization, a GiGi's Playhouse, or an informal parent group, it is a great idea for you to get connected and find out more information about what the group can offer. Groups can offer your family a chance to meet and connect with other families who have some shared life experiences. Over the years, those families can serve as a resource to one another. Groups may also offer classes or events to get involved in the local community.

GiGi's Playhouse

Nancy Gianni opened the first playhouse in Hoffman Estates, Illinois in 2003 after feeling led to do something for her daughter, GiGi, and change perceptions about Down syndrome. The goal was to provide a place for families to connect and find resources and support while networking with other families in the community. Today, there are more than 30 locations internationally that provide free educational and therapeutic programs to those with Down syndrome from birth to adulthood. To see if you have a local GiGi's or more information visit: *http://gigisplayhouse.org*.

OUR EXPERIENCE: Connecting Locally

My local DSA connects me to parents who understand my journey. The children in my local association are my child's friends—best friends. They help facilitate play groups and therapy to supplement every age group. Understanding that I was not alone in this journey has made such a difference to me. The Down Syndrome Association of the Brazos Valley shares life with us, and I am grateful for that.

—KELLEY JORDAN

They are more like a family than a group. One person's child is everybody's child. They offer support, acceptance, and advice completely free of judgment. With a new diagnosis they were invaluable to me in not only accepting what was to come but embracing it.

—HEATHER HOLBROOK

I love our mom's group. We get together once a month, and every time we get together I learn something about Down syndrome that I didn't know before. We just had a playdate and were sharing learning apps and tools. They all give the best advice.

—KATIE BEE

What We Do Locally

Parents who reach out to the Down Syndrome Guild (DSG) of Greater Kansas City, an effective, active local organization, following a prenatal or postnatal diagnosis are able to access a wealth of support during a critical time. A staff member will deliver a welcome basket full of books, videos, resources, and baby gifts to celebrate the baby's arrival. Parents are invited to attend quarterly support breakfasts where they will meet other parents who also have children up to two years of age. If their baby has any medical issues, parents can request DSG staff/volunteers to visit with them at the hospital, a goody bag of treats, and a $50 check to put toward a hospital stay overnight or longer. The guild provides a parent-to-parent match for members whose children have experienced similar medical issues. Referrals are provided for early intervention services and to connect with one of DSG's fourteen community groups, which operate under DSG's umbrella. Families receive support and connect with parents in their immediate geographic area through these programs. DSG provides information on the Ds health-care guidelines, lending library, sibling events, DSG Facebook groups, upcoming seminars and conferences, or social events on DSG's calendar. "Our goal," says Amy Allison, DSG executive director, "is to be a trusted partner, guidepost, and number one resource for families who have a loved one with Down syndrome."

Online Opportunities

The widespread use of technology has opened up a whole world of information and support to families with a child with Down syndrome. The information is a layer of support that families appreciate. More than the information, the connections families make online are invaluable. Many parents who may not have a local organization or access to other families find online groups and forums a lifeline of support during their children's lives.

OUR EXPERIENCE: Connecting Online

I could not imagine raising my child with Down syndrome without the Internet (Facebook, blogs, etc.). Help is available at the touch of a few keystrokes. I don't feel alone. I have met incredible "friends" around the world. I learn new things every day that will help me help my child. I am so grateful for Facebook and all the groups I am in. It is a tremendous source of support.

—CHRISTINE HAWKINS

The online support I found was the first actual "support" I accepted from anyone. I had a difficult time accepting words of wisdom and advice from family and friends who had no experience with special needs. The first time I chatted with a mom online who had a child with Ds, and she told me, "Things are going to be fine. He will truly be everything you wanted and more," was the first time I took a breath and really felt like someone understood. It was the ray of hope I desperately needed.

—SHANNON STASKIEWICZ

The online support is *amazing*. It's available twenty-four hours a day, connecting across the globe with other moms just like me who just get it. We get to go through the ups and downs of Down syndrome with each other without being judged and get to watch our beautiful children grow into their individual selves.

—ERIN STATZ

When Violette was born, the world of Down syndrome seemed like a huge, scary mystery. I felt very alone. I needed an outlet that would help me learn all that went with the extra chromosome that came with my beautiful girl. I had participated in an online mom group when I was pregnant with my oldest and that support was vital. I knew that with Violette, finding a safe place online where I could ask my questions any time of day (or middle of the night) would be key. Soon, I landed at BabyCenter's Down syndrome message board. I found real people—parents with children my daughter's age, along with wise mamas a few years ahead of me.

I asked questions, learned from moms, and got my head on straight when it came to what Down syndrome would mean to our family. The anonymity allowed me to be quite frank and blunt with all of my questions. Eight years later, as a group owner, I am offering support and connections and wisdom as an older mother. I have developed countless lifelong friendships all over the world. The life that seemed so isolating and lonely at first has been exactly the opposite.

—MISSY SKAVLEM

Early Intervention

Within the first weeks of the birth of your baby, you will be given information from the hospital or your pediatrician to meet with professionals in your local early intervention (EI) system. EI is a federally funded locally run program, in coordination with the school districts, which serves infants and children with disabilities and/or developmental delays until preschool (typically age three, depending on location). Generally, each child is assigned a case worker who will work with you to coordinate therapy services (physical, speech, occupational) and monitor the child's progress.

Updated in 2014, the U.S. Department of Education Office of Special Education Programs developed a resource for parents to better understand what EI is and how it can be a resource for families. This helpful overview is also available in Spanish. Early Intervention is a federal program that is accessed locally by parents through the local school district. All services are covered and aim to provide educational and developmental support for those who qualify.

EI focuses on these areas:

- Physical (reaching, rolling, crawling, walking)
- Cognitive (thinking, learning, solving problems)
- Communication (talking, listening, understanding)
- Social/emotional (playing, feeling secure and happy)
- Self-help (eating, dressing)

To meet these needs, EI offers services such as:

- Assistive technology (devices a child might need)
- Audiology or hearing services
- Speech and language services
- Counseling and training for your family
- Medical services
- Nursing services
- Nutrition services
- Occupational therapy
- Physical therapy
- Psychological services

Source: Center for Parent and Information Resources (*www.parentcenterhub.org/repository/ei-overview*)

Early Intervention for Your Child

"Often new parents don't realize that there is a federal law that assists them in getting the needed support and services for their infant and/or toddler. The Individuals with Disabilities Education Act (IDEA) contains a specific section, called Part C, that creates authority for states to set up coordinated systems of support for infants and toddlers with a diagnosis such as Down syndrome. Every state sets up its own system, but generally your doctor or your Down syndrome connections can help you to find out how to connect with the agencies that run your early intervention program.

"The law requires that services be delivered in a child and family's 'natural environment.' The intent of this provision is to ensure that the services make sense for children and families. Early intervention professionals are trained to deliver services in a way that integrates them into the regular routines followed by you and your child. You are the best person to know what that means for your child and family, and you will want to be an active member of your child's Individual Family Service Plan team." —Roxane Romanick, MSW

Individual Family Service Plan (IFSP)

Once you enter the early intervention program, the case worker will observe and evaluate your child and create a plan to best meet his or her needs. You'll look at this plan together with the EI team, sign off on it, and review it regularly. As described by the Center for Parent Information and Resources:

The IFSP is a written document that outlines the early intervention services that your child and family will receive. One guiding principal is that the family is a child's greatest resource, that a young child's needs are closely tied to the needs of his or her family. The best way to support children and meet their needs is to support and build upon the individual strengths of their family. So, the IFSP is a whole family plan with the parents as major contributors in its development. Involvement of other team members will depend on what the child needs. These other team members could come from several agencies and may include medical people, therapists, child development specialists, social workers, and others. More information on IFSP can be found in Chapter 6.

Source: *www.parentcenterhub.org/repository/ei-overview*

Therapists

Specialized therapists can help your child develop the communication, sensory, motor, and self-care skills needed for success throughout her life. To begin with, you'll typically work with speech, physical, and occupational therapists. All of you will work as a team to support your child's skill development. Some therapists coach the parent to be the teacher. Other therapy models focus on instruction from the therapist. Whichever model, it is important for you to work on skill development with your child outside of therapy times. Incorporating exercises into your baby's play is a natural way to accomplish this.

In addition to the state-provided services through early intervention, there are also private therapy options in many places. Your medical team can provide you with a list of resources in the area.

Getting to Know Your Therapists

As with any aspect of parenting, it's important that you understand what the different people who work with your child will do.

- A physical therapist (PT) will work to support your child in gross motor development. Some skills they will help your child with are rolling, sitting, crawling, standing, and walking.
- An occupational therapist (OT) will work to support daily living skills. They may focus on eating, dressing, bathing, and playing.
- A speech therapist (ST) or speech language pathologist (SLP) will help your child communicate, including both expressive (speaking) and receptive (listening) skills. Speech therapists can also help with feeding therapy if this is needed.

Development

As your child grows, he'll need help in physical skills, including gross motor development and fine motor skills. Down syndrome creates challenges in both these areas, but they are ones that—with the help of your medical team—your child can overcome.

From the PT—Gross Motor Development

"Low muscle tone is a characteristic of people with Down syndrome. Muscle tone is the natural tension in your muscle. Babies with low muscle tone may seem 'floppy,' as if they may slip through your hands when you pick them up. This cannot be changed because muscle tone is determined by genetics, but physical therapy can influence it by preventing poor posture and building core strength, for example. Parents can promote better posture by swaddling. This allows the baby to flex his or her muscles against the swaddle to help build strength. You can encourage good positioning by maintaining your baby's midline—the imaginary line drawn from the head to the feet separating the left and the right halves of the baby's body. Keep your baby's hands together or to his mouth and his head looking forward without a tilt. Tummy time is also very important from birth because it is the best way to build strength. Initially, tummy time can be done by placing the baby on mom or dad's chest, but eventually you should transition to the floor so your baby can work on more advanced skills such as rolling." —Kristi Allison, physical therapist

From the SLP—Speech Development

"The first six months of life are filled with milestones related to communication. Communication is the way your child hears, understands, and expresses. During the first three months your baby will begin to look at faces and smile at you. You may even hear a little giggle. Soon she will discover her voice and make sweet cooing sounds when you talk to her. As your baby gains head control she will start to turn her head toward your voice.

Hearing is essential for learning to talk. If your baby passed her newborn hearing screening, then the next hearing test should occur around six months of age. If she did not pass the screening, talk to your primary-care doctor about further testing.

More than anything, the first six months are important for bonding. Learn to read your baby's cues for hunger and discomfort. Notice the little things that make her happy. Whether this is your first baby or fourth, each child is different. Take the time to hug, kiss, snuggle, and get to know your baby." —Jennifer Bekins, Speech Language Pathologist

From the OT—Learning and Practicing New Skills

"The first six months of life is a time when your baby is learning some basic skills that he will perfect as he gets older.

- **Feeding.** This is a time for nourishment and oral motor development, as well as for holding, loving, and communicating with your child. Bonding and attachment is paramount to all development. Your baby may require intervention to assist with optimal positioning or perhaps exercises or equipment to help develop the ability to suck and swallow with efficiency and coordination. Because of low muscle tone in the lips, tongue, and jaw, children with Ds may have difficulty with the oral motor skills necessary to progress with textures and to develop efficient chewing skills. Children with Ds may also have sensory sensitivities to taste, texture, or temperature of food.

- **Play.** During play time, put your child in varying positions to help with motor control. We can't overemphasize the importance of tummy time. Babies with Down syndrome all have low muscle tone to some degree. It is very important for your baby to have frequent opportunities to work his muscles against gravity. This is best accomplished playing on the floor. Strong back and core muscles will enable your baby to learn to roll, sit, crawl, and pull to stand.
- **Bath.** Apart from being a fun time for you to watch your baby interacting with water, this is a time for sensory input through the tactile (touch) system, while playing and getting washed. A warm bath is calming and can help your baby relax and get ready for sleep." —Elaine Feingold-Toper, M.S., OTR/L and Cheryl Kurchin Chapman, MA, OTR/L

Future Planning and Support for Families

Because your child has Down syndrome, you may qualify for several federal and state programs available to help with finances and insurances. Check with your medical professionals, local organization, or EI team for more information specific to your state and visit the website of the PACER Center to review "Possibilities: A Financial Resource For Parents of Children with Disabilities" (*www.pacer.org/publications/possibilities*).

There may also be a waiver program for children with Intellectual Disabilities (ID) or Developmental Disabilities (DD) in your state. These programs are generally not income-based. For details, contact your state's Department of Health and Human Services.

OUR EXPERIENCE: State Waivers

After Noah was born, we knew we wouldn't qualify for any income-based support. We knew there were pieces of medical equipment that could support his learning and growth, but that it would be very costly. Our state offers another option, the Katie Beckett Waiver. This program can be used to pay for medically necessary services and equipment allowed under the Wisconsin Medicaid program. It uses the standards for disability under the Social Security Administration for children. We were able to use the waiver to help pay for items like glasses and SMO (ankle braces) without paying the full price out of pocket.

—JENNY DHEIN

Women, Infants, and Children (WIC)

WIC is an income-based resource available to families of children with Ds. This state-managed program provides support to moms and children with nutritious food, nutrition education and counseling, and screening and referrals to other health, welfare, and social services. You have to apply for the program, and it's given based on income standards at the state level. This program is intended to be used for a short time, and those who qualify are eligible for a specific certification period. Typically, WIC provides benefits to a family for six months to a year. To apply, visit *www.fns.usda.gov/wic/about-wic*.

Supplemental Security Income (SSI)

A child with a disability may also be eligible for SSI. This is a government program that helps to offset costs for families. SSI provides monthly payments to children and families with disabilities who qualify based on income and resources. To qualify, you need to apply and complete a Child Disability Report. Work with your area Social Security office to determine whether or not you're eligible. Your medical or EI team may also be able to offer guidance. For more information, visit *www.socialsecurity.gov*.

Medicaid

Because there are associated health conditions and concerns that may come along with Ds, it is important for your child to have medical coverage. Medicaid is a program that covers medical and health-care costs of people who qualify, including children up to age nineteen, pregnant women, and children with disabilities. There are a range of programs and services covered through Medicaid. This program works in conjunction with the Social Security Administration, and in some areas, the application process is the same. For details on applying in your state, visit the U.S. Department of Health and Human Services at *www.insurekidsnow.gov/state/index.html*.

OUR EXPERIENCE: Applying for Support

After Erin was diagnosed (prenatal diagnosis at about twenty weeks), one of my fears was all the medical issues and therapy she might have to have: PT, OT, speech, and who knows how many specialists she might need. Florida's Department of Children and Families (DCF) makes the process of applying for Medicaid very easy. I was able to do everything online and the case workers were so nice. They were patient and answered every question. I was able to see a great maternal-fetal medicine doctor that I never would have gotten into had DCF not helped me. They also helped me get a wonderful pediatrician who has experience with Ds children. I know my Erin can get great care because of the assistance they provide. One worry gone!

—CANDICE NUGENT

We were set up with the state resources through our NICU and the hospital's social worker. No red tape, no phone tag. All said and done before we left the hospital. Through all of Emilee's surgeries and treatments, it has definitely been a lifeline. I don't know how we would have made it through without it.

—JENNIFER KING

Planning for the Future

Due to income limits often associated with SSI and insurance coverage, families often need an alternative to provide some financial support for their child's future. While it may seem like a long way off, it is important to begin to think about the future and prepare. Consider drafting or redrafting your will to make sure your child is provided for in the event of your death. Discuss these options with your lawyer and/or financial advisor. You have several options.

1. **Special Needs Trust.** A special needs trust, or "supplemental care trust," is designed to support your child both before and after your death. The trust allows family and friends to gift your child monies without impacting her

benefits or eligibility for government programs or assistance. The trust also allows for you, as the parent, to establish guardianship and other important details about your child's future. It can be expensive to establish a special needs trust, and it is important to work with a lawyer who has experience in this area.

2. **Achieving a Better Life Experience (ABLE) account.** This federal legislation, passed in 2014, is another way for you to save for your loved ones with special needs. States are now in the process of working out the details for their citizens, and ABLE accounts should be widely available in the years to come. ABLE accounts work similarly to a traditional 529 college savings plan. The account is funded for and put into the name of the person with disabilities. Expenses that may be paid for through the ABLE accounts include housing, transportation, education, and medical/dental care. According to the National Down Syndrome Society's website, "The legislation also contains Medicaid fraud protection against abuse and a Medicaid pay-back provision when the beneficiary passes away. It will eliminate barriers to work and saving by preventing dollars saved through ABLE accounts from counting against an individual's eligibility for any federal benefits program."
3. **Letter of Intent.** A Letter of Intent (LOI) gives guidance, in the case of an emergency, that enables your family and friends, as well as the state, to know your intentions regarding your child. It is less intensive (and stressful) for parents to create, and provides information to help those who come after you about the needs of your offspring. Start simple; think about what a caregiver would need to know if you went out of town for a week and the day-to-day details that would make that week successful. The LOI should include:

- Your child's common daily routine, including details that are helpful such as "Prefers to take morning medicine with a glass of milk" and other simple tips that make life easier for your child and their caregiver while you are away.
- Diet considerations, allergies, and sensitivities; plus, again, likes and dislikes.
- Medical care information, list of doctors' names and phone numbers, regular appointment schedules, current medications and renewal notes, and medication allergies. (If you use the DS-Connect online resource, include the password to access your child's medical history. More on DS-Connect in Chapter 10.)
- Education, important goals, and Individualized Educational Plan (IEP) notes.
- Government benefits received by your child.
- Living arrangements (describe the current living arrangement and what the next-best alternative would be for your child, and why).
- Social information: clubs, likes, and friends.
- Religious information.

Then make a note of preferred long-term arrangements for your child. Since this is not a will, this documentation will be used as guidance only. Remember to update this document regularly.

OUR EXPERIENCE: The First Six Months

It took five months and two days for me to embrace Down syndrome. I accepted it about two months after our prenatal diagnosis, but embracing it was a different story.

The first month of Anderson's life, there were dark moments. How much would this disability actually disable him? But at six weeks he started to smile, [and] at ten weeks he started laughing

—which quickly became his favorite thing to do. He rolled over before he turned three months old.

He kept surprising me, surprising his therapists, surprising everyone.

And then at five months and two days *it* happened. It was the moment I dreaded as soon as we found out about the diagnosis. As I buckled Anderson into his car seat at a Panera, a woman with a wide smile and glasses came over to us.

She said, "He is just adorable." Then she said, "He has the most interesting almond-shaped eyes."

Gut check.

I had a choice. I could sidestep the issue and leave, or I could advocate for my son.

I said to her, "That's because he has Down syndrome." Her eyes got big behind her glasses. *I thought she knew*. She said, "But you look so young for *this* to happen to you."

My body temperature started rising, but I thought to myself: *Grace*. Give her grace, Jill. *After all, that's exactly what you thought when you got the diagnosis*.

She asked me when we found out. I told her halfway through the pregnancy. "Twenty weeks! Oh that's tough . . ." I started sweating because I knew what she was getting at. Then, Anderson started giggling. *Thank God*.

I looked at her with a smile and I said, "It wouldn't have changed anything had we found out earlier."

She asked me if I knew anything about his prognosis. I told her that just like all humans are born with different abilities and limitations, so are people with Down syndrome. But I added, "I know this boy is going to do amazing things." She smiled. Anderson smiled some more. And I couldn't stop smiling.

I smiled because I knew it was just the first of many hearts my son will change. I smiled because the thing I feared the most, the thing I thought would end life as I knew it . . . five months and two days later I could say, *I'm thankful for Down syndrome*.

—JILLIAN BENFIELD, BLOGGING AT
WWW.NEWSANCHORTOHOMEMAKER.COM

Resources

Finding Online Support

- BabyCenter—Down Syndrome Board: *http://community.babycenter.com/groups/a315/down_syndrome*
- Down Syndrome Diagnosis Network (DSDN): *www.dsdiagnosisnetwork.org*
- International Down Syndrome Coalition (IDSC): *http://theidsc.org/resources/support-for-parents.html*

Finding Medical Professionals

- Global Down Syndrome Foundation—Medical Centers: *www.globaldownsyndrome.org/research-medical-care/medical-care-providers*
- National Down Syndrome Society—U.S. Down syndrome clinic locations: *www.ndss.org/Resources/Health-Care/Health-Care-Providers*

For Planning for the Future

- PACER Center: *www.pacer.org/publications/possibilities/saving-for-your-*

childs-future-needs-part1.html

- ABLE Act: *www.ndss.org/Advocacy/Legislative-Agenda/Creating-an-Economic-Future-for-Individuals-with-Down-Syndrome*

For Early Intervention

- Parent Center Hub: *www.parentcenterhub.org/repository/ei-overview*
- Bruni, Maryanne. *Fine Motor Skills in Children with Down Syndrome: A Guide for Parents and Professionals*. Bethesda, MD: Woodbine House, 1998.
- Buckley, Sue, Emslie, M., Haslegrave, G., and LePrevost, P. *The Development of Language and Reading Skills in Children with Down's Syndrome*. Portsmouth, UK: The Sarah Duffen Centre, Portsmouth University, 1986.
- Kumin, Libby. *Early Communication Skills for Children with Down Syndrome: A Guide for Parents and Professionals*. Bethesda, MD: Woodbine House, 2003.
- Winders, Patricia. *Gross Motor Skills for Children with Down Syndrome: A Guide for Parents and Professionals*. Bethesda, MD: Woodbine House, 1997.

For Health

- Buckley, Sue. *Down Syndrome: Guidelines for Practice in Health Education and Social Care*. Oxford, UK: Blackwell Publishers, 2004.
- Skallerup, Susan. *Babies with Down Syndrome: A New Parents' Guide*. Bethesda, MD: Woodbine House, 2008.

Chapter Five
Six Months Through Two Years

Dear New Parent,

You made it!! The six-month mark is one to be celebrated for new families. Many of the initial doctor visits and appointments are wrapping up, and families tend to settle into patterns. Your baby is growing and changing in many wonderful ways. You have found a support team, including many local resources. Big things are ahead in the coming years and you've got a front-row seat.

How Do You Feel?

This is probably one of the most frequent questions you're asked by family, friends, and your medical support team. Sometimes, not daring to show weakness, you may reply, "Oh, fine! Great! Never better." But it's important to be honest with yourself and with your team. So how do you *really* feel?

Exhausted

Parents everywhere understand their common bond: exhaustion. Having a new child can be draining, both physically and emotionally, but when you add in all the unknowns and worry that come after a diagnosis of Down syndrome, your exhaustion is magnified. This might also be the time that your perfectly sleeping baby never wants to sleep. Ever. Or it might be the time that your poor sleeper finally starts to get a good stretch of sleep. And, finally, so do you. Taking care of yourself is important. Carving out a few minutes for you each day can go a long way to feeling more relaxed and rested. Consider taking a walk, doing yoga, or meditating.

Hopeful

The initial fear and worries of the first days, weeks, or months may have finally given way to thoughts of what the future holds for your child. As your baby interacts, grows, and begins to meet milestones, it may become much easier to relax. Although there will still be worry, it is tempered by the fact that you are getting to know your child and are able to see that, like other children, she will grow and develop and learn on her timetable. And you will get to watch those beautiful moments unfold.

Frustrated

Each child is different, and you may start to notice other children, with Ds or not, meeting milestones more quickly than your child. You may be anxiously awaiting several firsts with your baby and wondering if they will ever happen. Many parents feel this way. After many months of appointments and therapies, it is sometimes difficult to be patient in awaiting results.

Confident

Now that you have a team of support in place and have a solid background of information, you may feel ready to conquer the world! You may be thinking about awareness, advocacy, and getting involved in a Down syndrome organization, locally or nationally.

OUR EXPERIENCE: Six Months In

I'm in love. I didn't think I would be a good enough mother but Princess has shown me so much.

—MONIQUE FORYA

Eight months and I'm loving every second of being Lily's mum. Rolling, sitting up, feeding herself, drinking from a cup, starting to try and crawl, saying "Dadda." She is exceptional and makes my heart hurt with pride every day!

—VICKI BEDELL

Bradyn is eight and a half months, and I love it. He is changing and developing every day. Though to be honest, I have been having a hard time lately with seeing his peers starting to pull themselves to standing, while Bradyn is still working on unsupported sitting.

—HEATHER ASCHERIL

After six months I finally realize, I had a baby. Not a baby with Down syndrome or a baby with health risks, but a happy little baby boy. He's the light of my life and I wouldn't have it any other way!

—ALICE FLUHRER

We are simply happy to be eating. Life post–heart surgery is a different world, and we are so glad to be here.

—ELIZABETH JEUB

Acceptance

It may take time to understand and accept that your baby has Down syndrome. Certainly there are parents who don't think twice after hearing the diagnosis, and there are those who take years before really coming to terms with it. Some parents describe acceptance as a form of the grieving process, while others never really think about Ds. It is important to process the information and work through it on your own timeline. Whether it is your friends, family, a counselor, or a therapist, many parents find that talking about their questions, concerns, and fears helps through the beginning stages of a new diagnosis.

OUR EXPERIENCE: Moving Forward

We received an at-birth diagnosis, so obviously no one could say 100 percent immediately that Nora had Down syndrome, and it came as quite a shock initially, but when we finally received the positive T21 result, I think both my husband and I instantly accepted it. When we see Nora, we don't see Down syndrome, we see our daughter, and she is perfect.

—BETH KAZMIERCZAK

It was really important to me that I was happy on the day of the girls' birth. While I had worked through a lot of feelings on my own, I still had some thoughts and feelings that made me feel guilty, and that I just didn't really want to share with friends or family. I actually went to a therapist for the last two months of my pregnancy so that I could get it all out. It actually worked out very well and I felt much better once I was able to say what I needed to with no judgment and know that those things stayed there in that office.

—PAIGE BRADLEY

Acceptance came when I went to a play titled *Rare* that starred nine adults with Ds. It was a docudrama, so it was a play about their lives and their experience as people who happen to have Ds. I saw nine very different people. A gay man. A woman who spoke nine languages. And more. They felt a full range of emotions and had very distinct personalities. What happened

> for me was I began to see Tyler as more than a medical diagnosis and a list of potential medical problems. He became my son—a person first—and I wondered what he would be like as he grew up. What would his hopes and dreams be? My job suddenly became about ensuring that Tyler had all the tools to live a joyful and fulfilled life and to try and remove any barriers.
>
> —VALERIE TIH

Sharing Your Experience

Many families use writing as a tool to express themselves. Through blogs, websites, and Facebook pages, parents are able to share their experiences with Down syndrome and their family life. This sharing of information has allowed new parents to gain a much greater glimpse into life with Down syndrome. Photos, milestones, life: It is all there for others to see and learn from. Holly Christensen, blogging at whoopsiepiggle.com, writes:

> As a writer, I process everything through writing. I started my blog in October 2012, two months after Lyra's birth, and soon found having a virtual audience made me write regularly. Many of my essays have been about Ds and my unfolding understanding of what it means to be a person with Ds, both physically (more positive than I previously believed) and societally (how widely held misperceptions of Ds commensurately affect opportunities). The more I learned and wrote, the more I thought there needs to be a book for people who do *not* know someone with Ds. I'm a big open-minded liberal who had shockingly little accurate info on Ds. Nor had I thought much about Ds before Lyra. I want to change everyone else's perspective and make the world a more hospitable and

healthy place where my daughter can live, work, and play to her fullest. You know, change the world by eradicating old and false notions of Ds. Clearly I am not alone in this mission and this is just my hopeful contribution.

Meriah Nichols began blogging about her perspective on life with a disability and raising a child with Down syndrome. Meriah is a deaf woman, and writing provided an outlet for sharing her thoughts and stories with a wider audience. Blogging at *A Little Moxie*, she aims to share what life is really like for their family. "I did blog before I had Moxie, but I started to get real and honest after she came," she writes. Meriah also collects other families' stories of their experience with Down syndrome and hosts a comprehensive list of bloggers about Ds on her site. To follow her story and to find additional blogs focused on Down syndrome and disability, visit *www.meriahnichols.com*. Also check out more details in Chapter 11.

Milestones

When will the next milestone happen? Whether it is the long-awaited smile, those first rolls, a scoot across the floor, or those triumphant beginning steps, the firsts for a child are an occasion for celebration. It may take much longer than a parent expects, but many parents feel it makes it even better when it finally does happen. Each child, like any other, accomplishes tasks on his or her own timeline. Every child excels in some areas and may need support in others. Following is a chart of several common milestones. Review further guidelines through the Down Syndrome Medical Interest Group based in the UK at *www.dsmig.org.uk*.

MILESTONE COMPARISON CHART			
Area	**Milestone**	**Range for Children with Down Syndrome**	**Typical Range**
Gross Motor	Sits Alone	6–30 Months	5–9 Months
Gross Motor	Crawls	6–30 Months	5–9 Months
Gross Motor	Stands	1–3.25 Years	8–17 Months
Gross Motor	Walks Alone	1–4 Years	9–18 Months
Language	First Word	1–4 Years	9–18 Months
Language	Two-Word Phrases	2–7.5 Years	15–32 Months
Social/Self-Help	Responsive Smile	1.5–5 Months	1–3 Months
Social/Self-Help	Finger Feeds	10–24 Months	7–14 Months
Social/Self-Help	Drinks From Cup Unassisted	12–32 Months	9–17 Months
Social/Self-Help	Uses Spoon	13–39 Months	12–20 Months
Social/Self-Help	Bowel Control	2–7 Years	16–42 Months
Social/Self-Help	Dresses Self Unassisted	3.5–8.5 Years	3.25–5 Years

Source: Courtesy of the National Down Syndrome Society
(www.ndss.org/Resources/Therapies-Development/Early-Intervention)

View a text version of this table

OUR EXPERIENCE: Waiting on Milestones

When he finally smiled, it was the first time I felt like he was like any other baby. After feeding issues, a two-month hospital stay, and coming home on a heart monitor, it was a much-needed feeling of normal.

—JILL GRIFFITH

Her first smile and laugh. I needed those so terribly in those early days.

—VICKIE KOCHANS

Still waiting on talking . . . I think I was okay waiting for the walking part because I *knew* he would get there, whether it be by two, three, or even four or five; he would walk. You don't see adults with Ds struggling to walk (typically), but you see the struggle with words and communication.

—AMBER SMITH

Crawling. That was the one big thing I waited for. Once he crawled it allowed him to get around and explore more. Speech not so much because he's doing great with words and communicating. He is two and not walking independently yet but oh, so close.

—SHERYL SMITH

Sitting up. I felt like when she was able to sit up independently it would add a whole new dimension of playing. That was the hardest for us!

—JANESSA GROSS

Crawling was one I was anxious about. It was important to me that she learn to four-point crawl because research has shown it to be so beneficial to development.

—HEATHER BRADLEY

Walking. We thought once she was walking, that would mean she was on her own and wouldn't need to depend on us as much. It was a sign of real independence.

—LEYDA SIMON

For us, it was hardest to wait for speech. Renner is so vocal but doesn't have many formed words yet, and it's so hard as a parent when you know they are trying to communicate with you through their speech, but it just isn't there quite yet.

—KAREN WOLLMAN

Motor Skills

Walking and talking top the list of most anticipated milestones for parents. Gross motor development involves how a child uses all his large-muscle groups. NDSS provides several resources for parents in this area, including advice from Patricia C. Winders, Senior Physical Therapist, Down Syndrome Specialist, Sie Center for Down Syndrome, Children's Hospital, Aurora, CO. Winders states: "The goal of physical therapy for these children is not to accelerate the rate of their development, as is often presumed, but to facilitate the development of optimal movement patterns. This means that over the long term, you want to help the child develop good posture, proper foot alignment, an efficient walking pattern, and a good physical foundation for exercise throughout life." For more information, visit *www.ndss.org/Resources/Therapies-Development/Physical-Therapy-Down-Syndrome*.

Advice from the Physical Therapist

"The majority of children with Down syndrome meet their gross motor milestones—such as crawling and walking—but on their own timetable. And that's okay! More important than meeting skills at a certain age is learning to be independent and using good quality of movement. Be patient! Look for progress in terms of performing a skill with more confidence, more ease, or with less assistance. Most importantly, remember that *you* are the most important contributor to physical therapy success.

"Consider the number of waking hours your child has to work on attaining skills. Your physical therapist has very limited time to work with your offspring, so ask your PT to help you build opportunities into your child's daily routine. Work to educate every person in your child's life on how best to help. For example, if your child is practicing trunk rotation while sitting—rotating the upper body while his lower body stays stable—then teach siblings to place favorite toys to the sides to encourage reaching with rotation. If your child is learning to climb steps, encourage him or her to climb the last few steps every time he or she goes upstairs to nap and then eventually progress to climbing the full flight of stairs." —Kristi Allison, Physical Therapist

Speech

Speech is a highly anticipated milestone. Parents long for those first words. Because the range in which a first, clear word may be used and spoken in a phrase or sentence varies so widely, parents realize that they must have an arsenal of tools to use for communicating. Your speech therapist or speech-language pathologist (SLP) will be an excellent resource. Whether you choose to use sign language, communication devices, or other tools, finding a way to communicate effectively and minimize frustrations is the key.

The NDSC provides resources prepared by Libby Kumin, PhD, CCC-SLP, at *www.ndsccenter.org/speech-and-language*. Here you will find communication resources for:

- The basis for speech
- First words and phrases
- Infants and toddlers
- Preschool through kindergarten
- Childhood apraxia
- School-age children
- Oral motor skill difficulties

Advice from the speech language pathologist

"Over the next eighteen months you will notice big changes in the way your child communicates. Your baby will begin to babble with repeated consonant sounds, like "da-da-da." After a while the babbling will change into jargon. Jargon has an adult-like rhythm, but is nonsense to the listener. Often parents say, "It sounds like she's talking in another language."

"When your baby learns to wave, she is beginning to understand that a gesture has meaning to others. It also means she is able to coordinate some movements of her arm and hand. These milestones are good indicators that she is ready to start simple sign language. The goal of signing is not to replace talking. Rather, signs are meant to bridge the gap until your child consistently uses single words to communicate with you. As she starts consistently talking to others, signs will fade from use.

"As your child gains more control over her head and arms, play games like peek-a-boo, rolling a ball, or tug of war with a favorite toy. These early games set the foundation for later conversational skills.

"Around eighteen months your child may start to say her first words. First words often resemble real words. For instance, your child may look at your dog and say, 'daw.' It is important to reinforce these attempts. Praise your baby for talking and repeat the word back to her. 'Dog! You're right! That's a dog.'" —Jennifer Bekins, SLP

Advice from the Occupational Therapist—Learning and Practicing New Skills

"Let's talk about meals. These are times to explore a variety of tastes and textures. Your child will be transitioning to solid foods. Some children with Down syndrome may be sensitive to new tastes and textures. Learning to eat table food may involve smaller increments of change, sensory strategies, time, and patience.

"Children in this age group are learning to use utensils and to drink from a cup. There are a variety of tools that can assist your child to develop grip strength and coordination as well as oral activities to help them use their lips and tongues effectively. One focus may be the use of a straw cup to assist in oral motor development.

"Another important activity in your baby's first six months is play. Play time is when your child moves and explores within her physical and social environment. Your child may be learning to walk, climb, and maneuver her body. Play outside! Your child is learning to use her hands as tools. She can develop skills with toys as well as everyday household items. Songs and games will help your child understand language and express herself through gestures, signs, or words.

"Finally, there's bath time. This is when your baby learns to undress, practice movement such as standing up and sitting down, identify body parts, and develop cognitive concepts such as in and out, hot and cold, empty and full." —Elaine Feingold-Toper, M.S., OTR/L and Cheryl Kurchin Chapman, M.A., OTR/L

Medical Care/Considerations

After the onslaught of appointments and checkups in the first six months of your child's life, medical care begins to fall to the background, depending on your child's needs. If your child has a heart defect, this may be the time that you are preparing for or recovering from open-heart surgery. It may be a time where you are working with your medical professionals to do further monitoring or testing in other areas like thyroid and hearing. There may also be other concerns you notice, like chronic congestion or delayed tooth eruption. It is important to continue to review the AAP Care

Guidelines at your child's appointments. Remember to continue to update your care notebook (Chapter 4). Let's turn now to some common medical/physical issues you may face after your child has passed six months.

Heart Surgery

If you fall into the 50 percent of families whose child with Down syndrome has a heart defect, you may be preparing for open-heart surgery (OHS). Although not all heart defects require surgery, many do. Along with information from your medical team, there are great resources available for you online to help navigate the process. Leah Thompson, blogging at Our Cora Bean, has collected family accounts and offers first-hand advice on preparing for surgery. She suggests:

- Read about the details of the defect, what the repair entails, what the possible complications are.
- Ask questions of your medical team before, during, and after the surgery.
- Read about other people's experiences; blogs are a wonderful resource—but remember, your experience will be your own!
- Prepare yourself with post-operation details and photos.
- Talk to your family and friends about the surgery.
- Ask your friends and family for help.

OUR EXPERIENCE: Hospital Stay Advice

Trust your instincts. You know your baby best, so speak up if you feel that something's not right during recovery, whether it's about controlling pain or noticing out-of-the-ordinary behavior. Since Cora's pain meds were discontinued less than forty-eight hours post-surgery and she seemed to be in quite a bit of pain, we took it upon ourselves to keep track of all her pain medication doses. And we'd page the nurses when her meds were due again. Definitely speak up if something feels wrong to you.

Rest. If you can, try and rest. Sleep while your baby sleeps, especially in the hours immediately after surgery (if you can). Take shifts by the bedside so you can step away here and there, and if you're comfortable with it, get out for a walk or a meal while a trusted friend or family member sits with your baby.

If you're not local: Ask about your local Ronald McDonald House or if there is a place to stay while your child is in the hospital. Many parents swear by having a "home" away from the hospital. I didn't leave the hospital myself. Most hospitals will provide you with a cot and some have a parents' room when your child is in the ICU. Perhaps I would have slept better in my own bed, but it's hard to say. I didn't get much sleep in the days prior, during, or after the surgery. Hopefully you'll fare better [than] I did in the sleep department.

—LEAH THOMSON, BLOGGING AT *WWW.OURCORABEAN.BLOGSPOT.COM*

Aspiration

Although reflux and gastroesophageal reflux disease (GERD) can be common in children with Down syndrome and do not always cause problems, weakness in the pharyngeal (throat) muscles can cause aspiration, which in turn can be a cause of some feeding and/or lung issues. Aspiration occurs when a child is swallowing and the drink or food travels down the trachea, rather than the esophagus. These substances can travel through the airway and settle in the child's lungs, sometimes resulting in pneumonia. If your child exhibits the following symptoms while eating or has recurrent pneumonia, you and your medical team may have to undertake a swallow study to gain more information.

- Bluish discoloration of the skin caused by lack of oxygen
- Chest pain
- Coughing up foul-smelling, greenish, or dark phlegm (sputum) or phlegm that has pus or blood
- Fatigue
- Fever
- Shortness of breath
- Wheezing
- Breath odor
- Excessive sweating
- Problems swallowing

Source: *www.nlm.nih.gov/medlineplus/ency/article/000121.htm*

OUR EXPERIENCE: Swallow Study and Aspiration

We have had three swallow studies done. The first was at four months as aspiration was suspected because of pneumonia present in her right upper lobe (the first place aspirated liquid would drain to). Baby was not allowed to eat for four hours prior in hopes to arrive hungry. She was placed in a reclined seat and fed a few sips of different [thicknesses] of formula from a bottle. The bottle also contained barium so as she was swallowing the doctors could watch in live motion through an x-ray machine.

The swallow study is kind of an experiment as thicknesses and bottle nipples with different flow rates are increased until one is properly swallowed. We had two additional studies at seven and twelve months to help plan for her feedings. We ended up thickening her liquids and that has helped a lot!

—JOY GRIFFIN

Infantile Spasms

Infantile spasms (IS) are a form of epilepsy that affect up to 13 percent of the Down syndrome population. If you suspect unusual behavior or seizure-like activity in your child, it is important to talk to a doctor. The only way to diagnose or rule out IS is through an exam and electroencephalography (EEG). If your child suffers from IS, the doctor usually will see an unusual pattern, called hypsarrhythmia, when the seizures are not occurring. This chaotic, high-voltage pattern is often helpful in confirming the diagnosis, according to the Epilepsy Foundation.

The Global Down Syndrome Foundation (GDSF) explains, "While infantile spasms are serious, they are not common. Children with infantile spasms stop progressing toward developmental milestones and may lose motor skills they have already mastered, such as sitting up or crawling. They may experience cognitive and speech regression as well. Unaddressed infantile spasms may permanently impair functionality and impact children's abilities—a serious concern for children with Down syndrome who may already have developmental delays."

The Epilepsy Foundation notes the following about IS:

- A seizure consists of a sudden jerk followed by stiffening.
- Each seizure lasts only a second or two but usually in a series.
- They are most common just after waking up and rarely occur during sleep.
- They typically begin between three and twelve months of age and usually stop by the time the child is four years old.
- Steroid therapy and the anti-seizure medicine Sabril are the primary treatments.
- Most children with IS are developmentally delayed later in life.
- Many children with Ds develop other kinds of epilepsy.

Sources: *www.globaldownsyndrome.org/sie-center-for-down-syndrome-takes-on-infantile-spasms*, *www.epilepsy.com/learn/types-epilepsy-syndromes*

OUR EXPERIENCE: Diagnosing Infantile Spasms

My son, Luca, started having these subtle jerking motions, and I wasn't sure if they were just immature baby reflexes, or something more. Within days, he started having them more regularly, in clusters, and they were getting more exaggerated. I had read about infantile spasms (IS), and had a gut feeling that was what was going on. I took him to the emergency room at the children's hospital with video of the episodes I had captured with our phones. The ER physician assured me that he was okay and that the jerking movements were benign. I was stunned, but didn't know what else to do, so I took him home.

The next day the episodes increased in frequency and intensity, and I was persistent with my pediatrician that she needed to see him. She saw the episodes and immediately admitted him to the hospital for an EEG. I learned that an EEG is the only true way to make the diagnosis. Within a few hours the neurologist was able to see that Luca's brain was in hypsarrhythmia, a distinct background wave pattern that is a hallmark sign of IS.

—JENNY DI BENEDETTO

What to Do If You Think Your Child Has IS

1. Know what IS looks like. This website has helpful information and a video showing two examples of an episode: *www.infantilespasmscenter.org*.
2. Be persistent in demanding that your pediatrician schedule an EEG to diagnose or rule out IS. Because IS is so rare, many physicians will never see it in their career.
3. Be as aggressive as possible with treatment. It's important to future development to stop the spasms as soon as possible.

4. Find a network that can support you. There are several Facebook pages aimed to help families of children with IS:

www.facebook.com/groups/infantilespasmscommunity
www.facebook.com/groups/ketogenicparents
For both of these, you will need to log into Facebook.

OUR EXPERIENCE: Treating Infantile Spasms

There are two pharmaceutical treatments that are approved by the FDA for IS and many others that are approved for epilepsy that physicians try based on their experience. They all come with significant side effects and risks, and making a decision on what to try first can be overwhelming. We started Luca on treatment immediately, and while many children with Down syndrome respond quickly to medication (within a few weeks), our son did not. He also started to have different types of seizures. As his case became more complicated over several months, we sought out a pediatric epileptologist (a neurologist who specializes in treating children with epilepsy) to treat him. We tried several different medications and the ketogenic diet (a high-fat low-carb diet used to treat epilepsy), and after what seemed like an eternity, we finally were able to stop the spasms, and return his brain pattern back to normal. He has resumed his developmental progress, and is back to his happy, interactive self.

—JENNY DI BENEDETTO

Head, Ankle, and Hip Supports

Due to decreased muscle tone, some children with Down syndrome may need additional physical supports as they develop and grow.

Head-Neck

Weak or loose neck muscles can be an area of concern for some children with Ds. Car seat support is important for all children and proper neck support for those with Ds is all the more important. Parents should also consider extended rear-facing for their child with Down syndrome to ensure additional support in the case of an accident. Some children develop flat spots on their heads due to increased time lying on their backs. This can be especially true for those that are in the NICU or hospital for an extended stay. Physical therapy and helmets can be used to help treat the flat spot and ensure future proper head shape and neck strength. Talk with your medical team for recommendations and referrals if you have concerns.

Ankle-Foot

Low muscle tone can also impact a child's stability in learning to stand-up and walk. Your physical therapist and pediatrician are great resources to talk about supports, like orthosis, that might help your child. Ankle-foot orthosis (AFOs) are braces, generally made of plastic, that are worn inside a shoe to add stability to a child's ankles/leg. There are other options, like *supra-malleolar orthosis* (SMOs) that also provide bracing support, but target different parts of the foot. If needed, your child will be fitted for the bracing and prescribed a schedule for wearing them. Physical therapists will help make the best decision about the best supports for your child's specific needs.

OUR EXPERIENCE: Orthotics

We got orthotics after an orthopedist and physical therapist recommended them for our daughter who was not yet standing independently or walking at two and a half years old. They were recommended to improve her ankle pronation and decrease the instability in the ankles that would cause her to lock her knees. It didn't take long for her to adjust to them and after only a few days she was standing for several seconds. She continues to improve daily with her gross motor skills.

—JAIME ERICKSON

Hips and Joints

According to Dr. Len Leshin, "Almost all of the conditions that affect the bones and joints of people with Down syndrome arise from the abnormal collagen found in Down syndrome. Collagen is the major protein that makes up ligaments, tendons, cartilage, bone, and the support structure of the skin. One of the types of collagen (type VI) is encoded by a gene found on the twenty-first chromosome. The resulting effect in people with DS is increased laxity, or looseness, of the ligaments that attach bone to bone and muscle to bone. The combination of this ligamentous laxity and low muscle tone contribute to orthopedic problems in people with Down syndrome."*www.ds-health.com/ortho.htm*.

Looser joints can lead to a greater chance of hip or knee problems for your child with Ds. Your pediatrician will examine your child for this during well-child checkups and your physical therapist can monitor for concerns too. You can be proactive by holding/carrying your child in a way that keeps hips together rather than splayed apart. Some parents use "hip helpers," a pair of shorts that work to keep the hips and legs closer together, as a way to treat loose hips.

OUR EXPERIENCE: Hip Dysplasia

Not all hip dysplasia is discovered in newborn screenings. Sometimes it can even take up to a year to develop and can be missed. I was glad I listened to Russell's body and what it was telling me when he started limping at age fourteen. Listen to your gut, heart, and child. It took us three different doctors and opinions to feel comfortable with a surgeon because of the seriousness of the surgery. We made sure Russell was in the best hands with a doctor and he was!

—ADRIENNE BIEVENUE

Micropenis

When a baby boy with Down syndrome is born, parents and doctors may notice he has a small penis. This is not uncommon and there are treatments available. It's important to diagnose, though, because it can occur in conjunction with other problems, particularly hormone disorders that, if they aren't treated, can disrupt the development of your child's sexual organs.

Doctors will diagnose a micropenis after they conduct a physical examination, including measurements. If a micropenis is suspected, you may be referred to a pediatric urologist (specializing in the male genital tract) or endocrinologist (specializing in hormones).

OUR EXPERIENCE: Asking for Answers

"Should I be concerned about the size of my son's penis?" [was] a thought that frequently crossed my mind. He was about six months old when I began noticing the lack of growth. It wasn't something I felt comfortable researching or talking about, and it was difficult to actually express concern to the pediatrician. I mentioned it to my son's pediatrician at his six-month well check, and the question was completely avoided. I let it go at the time but knew I needed to ask. We asked at the next well-child appointment and it was avoided again. At about twenty months we met with an endocrinologist who was willing to acknowledge our concern. She examined him and acknowledged that my suspicions were correct and my son had fallen behind on the penile growth scale. I was relieved, and we immediately began speaking about treatment. We decided to do testosterone therapy in the form of three monthly intramuscular injections to increase his penis size. Within a few weeks we were able to see [a] difference in the size, and a growth spurt was very obvious. No side effects had presented, and after the second dose, there was no longer a concern.

—JENNY WARD-CULKINS

Teeth

Children with Down syndrome may have additional dental considerations and needs. Generally speaking, you may notice teeth take longer to come in. Your child might not get his first teeth until he's close to turning one, and it could take up until his second birthday. When they do pop up, they may not be in the usual order. The teeth may also be smaller and sharper than a typical child's teeth. The AAP recommends a visit to the dentist within six months after the first tooth erupts or by one year of age. You can find additional information at *www.ndss.org/Resources/Health-Care/Associated-Conditions/Dental-Issues-Down-Syndrome*.

Sleep

In its updated care guidelines for those with Down syndrome, the AAP recommended in 2011 that parents schedule a sleep study for their children by age four. If your child has abnormal sleep patterns, you need to consult your pediatrician. A sleep study can provide you and your medical team more information about your child's breathing and sleep and determine whether additional oxygen may or may not be needed for your child. For some children who struggle with a form of apnea (that is, the interruption of normal breathing patterns when they sleep), your doctor may remove adenoids and tonsils to help. Other children may begin oxygen therapy in the form of continuous positive airway pressure (CPAP). Treating apnea allows for your child to have a more restful sleep and can lead to increased cognitive function.

Source: *http://aapnews.aappublications.org/content/early/2011/07/25/aapnews.20110725-3.full?rss=1*

Leukemia

Your doctor will monitor your child's bloodwork at well-child visits. Infants who had transient myeloproliferative disorder (TMD) have a greater chance of developing acute myeloid leukemia (AML). Children with Down syndrome have a greater chance of developing AML, but they also respond very well to the treatments. Symptoms to watch for, according to *www.stjude.org*, include:

- Fever
- Infection
- Easy bruising and bleeding
- Frequent nosebleeds
- Bleeding that is hard to stop, even from a small cut
- Pain in bones or joints
- Swollen glands
- Poor appetite

OUR EXPERIENCE: AML after TMD

Just after Camden's first birthday we discovered his platelet count had dropped drastically. He also had petechiae (small red blood spots) all over his body. He had had hand-foot-and–

mouth [disease, and] the doctors reassured us that it was just a reaction to that virus. Because he had TMD at birth, they watched him closely. Platelets continued to drop and by November his platelets were very low. He was always sleepy, and his appetite was diminished. We decided to do a bone marrow biopsy, and Camden was diagnosed with AML. We were told we would spend most of six to eight months in the hospital getting treatment.

I watched my sweet baby have his first chemo treatment. I expected him to wither and to regress from all the progress we had made, but children are so resilient. We were told that children with Down syndrome do better with chemo; the extra chromosome is more receptive. Some treatments have gone really well, and some have not. I quit my job as a critical care nurse to sit in with my baby day in and day out, days filled with treatments, blood draws, physical therapy, occupational therapy, speech therapy, doctors, CNAs, nurses, vital signs, chemo, uncomfortable beds . . .

I have become closer to everyone around me including my son. He has thrived in his surroundings. He has reached milestones faster and hasn't missed a beat. I have made friends I would never have had. I have seen more kindness than I ever thought possible. Camden's prognosis is good. To me he is perfect. I would go through all of this again to know that he is going to be okay. He is the best thing that ever happened to me. I love him more than ever; my heart fell apart and Camden is holding the pieces together.

—MEGHAN ROBERSON

Nutrition

It is important for every child, regardless of the number of chromosomes she has, to have a balanced diet that will support her physical and mental well-being. For children with Down syndrome, there are varying beliefs about what an appropriate diet includes. Some parents choose to supplement with additional vitamins. It is important to discuss questions and concerns with your medical team and seek out information.

The Right Tools

Your occupational or speech therapist may be able to help provide information, feedback, or resources if you are struggling with feedings. For example, straws and open cups help with oral development for children with Down syndrome, so they are often a better choice than a bottle or sippy cup. If you have concerns, contact your local speech or occupational therapist.

OUR EXPERIENCE: Straw Cup

At nearly three, Renner has been doing the TalkTools (TT) program (see the following for more information) for quite a long time now . . . they actually started in the NICU using the Z-Vibe tool when he was off life support and was stable enough. The Z-Vibe worked wonders in helping him not have an oral aversion. The straw cup has helped with proper tongue placement and work on oral motor skills . . . such as lip rounding. Renner has gained awesome lip closure now with working on the straws. The TT hierarchy of straws helps by working on teaching the tongue muscle to retract and will thus help with eating correctly and with speech.

—KAREN WOLLMAN

TalkTools

Sara Rosenfeld-Johnson founded TalkTools (TT) as an approach to serving those with speech, oral placement, and feeding disorders. TT offers assessment and therapy along with products to provide the best possible outcomes. Traveling clinics are provided to best serve those around the world with the hierarchical approach to oral placement therapy. Find out more online at *www.talktools.com*.

More Children

For some parents, having a child with Down syndrome does not change anything in their future parenthood plans. Some parents choose to expand their family further so their child will have a playmate to learn and socialize with or to support him in the future. Some parents choose to adopt another child with Down syndrome. If you decide on another child, perhaps you think differently about prenatal testing (assuming you didn't have it done the last time).

OUR EXPERIENCE: On Having More Children

Ds wasn't going to stop our family from growing! We wanted four and ended with three. Russell was our second. No fears, no nothing. We wanted kids!

—ADRIENNE BIEVENUE

We originally only wanted one child. When E was born and diagnosed, and I started doing research, I found out that kiddos with Ds lived well into their sixties or seventies. We decided to try for another. We figured E would outlive us old farts and he'd need a partner in crime. E was a game changer for us when it came to family planning.

—CARA JACOCKS

Since I'm a translocation carrier, we waited until we felt ready to have another child with Ds. I am super close with my brother, and we wanted Rowenna to have a chance at a sibling relationship like that. So far, looks good.

—MELISSA STOLTZ

We would like to add one more but hubby and I are both scared too.

—BRANDI LEMAY

We thought we were done until we met Dr. Jeannie Visootsak, former medical director at Emory University's Ds clinic. She was very encouraging when we expressed our concerns with having a second child. She suggested that having another child in the home might challenge and motivate Lucas to excel. She also cited that individuals and siblings reported being very happy to have each other and that their lives are enriched by having a sibling to care about and enjoy the company of.

—BRANDY SNOW

OUR EXPERIENCE: Testing the Next Time Around

Since the quad was "negative" and no ultrasound markers ever surfaced, I had mentally and emotionally "checked off" Down syndrome as something I should worry about. Looking back I wish we would have never done prenatal testing. At least I would have gone into delivery knowing it could be a possibility. I kept saying to my doc after she announced her suspicions, "But his test results were negative, right?" I think those inaccurate test results prolonged our acceptance of the diagnosis too. I really despise those tests on many levels. I had no idea that parents would terminate in some cases if the results were positive. We just wanted to prepare when we chose the quad screen with Everett. We were never given that opportunity. I refused testing with this current pregnancy because of the inaccuracy of our last test . . . that, and it just doesn't matter anymore. We'll take what God gives us and be happy. My mantra on those tests—fool me once, shame on you. Fool me twice, shame on me. I won't be blindsided again by one of those tests.

—CARA JACOCKS

I needed to know during my next pregnancy. After a birth diagnosis, I knew that I wanted to be prepared for anything this time around.

—JENNY DI BENEDETTO

Taking Action

Having a child with Down syndrome sometimes propels people to "do something." Whether that is parents reaching out to other new parents, sharing about their experience, spreading awareness, or advocating for legislation, there are many ways for parents to get involved, if they are interested.

OUR EXPERIENCE: Taking Action

During a brief stay at the Children's Hospital of Philadelphia (CHOP) for our infant son's open-heart surgery, we met many families who had also traveled to CHOP to get their children the best care possible. Under the heavy weight of caring for a sick child, we saw families becoming financially devastated by the burden of travel expenses they were incurring to be with their child, far from home. Understanding that health insurance doesn't cover the cost of travel for medical care, we decided to create Eli's Heart to help support families in need.

Sometimes the request is as simple as a mother needing gas cards to travel daily to see her child in a hospital three hours from home. Other times, we meet families who need assistance with airfare, lengthy hotel stays, [or] meals. The requests vary, but each story touches us deeply. We are proud to be a part of the Down syndrome community supporting fellow parents in their time of need and hope that these small acts of kindness can remove some of the stress and pressure of caring for a sick child.

—MELISSA AND CASEY CRAIG, FOUNDERS OF ELI'S HEART (*HTTP://ELISHEART.ORG*)

As Reeve grew, I thought a lot about the world around him. When I looked at Down syndrome and what the public does/doesn't know about it, I felt like one area that was really missing was to convey the love, fun, pride, and "normalness" that families who have a child with Down syndrome feel. I wanted to capture those feelings and help to reframe Down syndrome for people who are less familiar with it. I sensed that a lot of people found it uncomfortable—they didn't know whether or not to feel sorry for a family who had a child with Down syndrome. We were at the point of having a sense of humor and appreciation about it, so I wanted to "rebrand" it in a way. Delicate humor tends to be a good way to help people approach a topic that is normally very difficult to talk about, [and] I felt that careful humor—humor that celebrated and uplifted—could be very positive and make Down syndrome awareness and acceptance more approachable goals for the everyday person who may have otherwise been afraid of it.

—SHANA ANDERSON, FOUNDER OF REEVES TEES, *WWW.REEVESTEES.COM*

OUR EXPERIENCE: From Heart Surgery to School

Holding a baby after open-heart surgery is awkward. The sternum is cracked to give the doctors access to the heart, which means that lifting a child under the armpits isn't permitted. Enter car seats, cribs, swings, Bumbo seats, and any other place you might set a baby. Getting the child seated isn't a problem. Getting her back out is a pain.

I celebrated my first daughter's six-month birthday holding her awkwardly, shortly after she was released from the hospital following open-heart surgery. We kept a low profile to avoid germs.

Two years later, she walked into school with a backpack twice her size. She passed mommy, who was a teacher at her school, in the hallway and couldn't be bothered to say hi, because she was busy with her classmates.

By three, she would become a force of nature, keeping her family on their toes.

Transitioning from babyhood to toddlerhood with Ellie seemed to take forever. Although she signed and crawled at ten months, her first words were at eighteen months, and she bear crawled from her first birthday until she was two and a half. Yet her personality matched her typical toddler friends, demanding unreasonable things and changing her mind, throwing seemingly random tantrums followed by hugs and kisses.

The questions people ask during those transition years are hard for parents whose child has delays.

Is she walking? No. No. No. Still no.

Talking? Signing. Some. A little.

At six months, that medically fragile open-heart surgery survivor was markedly different from her peers. At two and a half, unsteady on her feet, strangers assumed Ellie was much younger. I sometimes was uncertain about my place—I needed to provide Ellie with physical assistance but I wanted her to soar independently.

Time passed. Her health improved.

And those milestones came with celebrations. She talked. She put two words together. She learned her ABCs. She took two steps . . . and a few months later, four steps . . . and a few months later, she began to walk.

She transitioned after two and a half years from receiving services in the safety of our own home to a five-hour, five-day-a-week school program provided by the county. I couldn't watch her therapies anymore. I didn't talk to her therapists very often compared to when they visited our house. I had to trust strangers with my baby and assume that she would grow and learn and be okay.

She soared. And I learned that those strangers were worth trusting, and would return my daughter to me at the end of each day more talkative, more adaptable, and with more skills than I imagined. More importantly, I learned that my girl would be happy at school, ready to take on the world even outside of our safe home.

—MEGAN LANDMEIER, BLOGGING AT *WWW.MYSTUBBORNMISS.COM*

Resources

For Your Information

- TalkTools: *www.talktools.com*
- Signing Time: *www.signingtime.com*
- Milestone Information: *www.dsmig.org.uk*
- IDSC groups for preschool–adult children: *http://theidsc.org/resources*
- Early Intervention Support: *www.parentcenterhub.org/repository/ei-overview*

Chapter Six
Ages Three Through Five

Milestones are being met and your child is growing and learning each day! Daily life is less full of therapies and appointments as you prepare for life's next transition: preschool! This may also be the time you seek out additional opportunities for your child in the form of sports, dance, or other activities. It is also likely you will venture into the world of potty training, depending on your child's readiness. Big things are happening for your toddler as he becomes a preschooler!

Dear Parent,

We're sure you are noting how quickly the time has passed by since the newborn days. Your child has grown in wonderful ways. She or he is communicating with you in some form, and your toddler is surely showing his or her personality as he or she prepares for entering school. The days of therapists in your home are maybe giving way to more structured learning and social environments. Enjoy watching your child continue to learn, excel, and grow!

Transition to School

Preschool! Most families are provided therapies in a home setting for the first years. When your child starts to attend school, state-funded therapy sessions may become a part of her school day. Some families may continue or add private therapy support as well, depending on their child's needs. Contact your local school district, EI team, and Down syndrome organization for more information. It will also be the time your Individual Family Service Plan (IFSP) probably transitions into an Individualized Education Plan (IEP). There will be lots of new (and exciting) changes in the years to come!

OUR EXPERIENCE: Transition to Preschool

Transitioning from early intervention to preschool was one of the scariest things we ever had to do. I couldn't protect him in school. Would he be accepted? Would they like him? Would he be treated fairly? We were scared; I cried! However, it was one of the best things that ever happened to him. He loved it! His IEP went well and his team that worked with him was phenomenal!

—BONNIE SCOTT

OUR EXPERIENCE: Considering Options

I had been on the fence about my daughter Moxie attending a traditional school. I'm sure the fact that I myself had a fluid educational experience, with a mix of homeschooling, unschooling, [and] public, parochial, and prep schools had something to do with it. The fact that I am a trained teacher had something to do with it, too. But when Moxie had a negative experience with her IEP meeting when she was three years old, I was pushed off the fence and into the homeschooling camp. I was absolutely not going to put her through that again, and I did not want to have my daughter boxed by what others might think she was lacking in. I did not want Down syndrome to define her; I wanted her to define Down syndrome. What I mean by that is, Down syndrome provides my daughter with a particular view of life. It's her lens through which she will view the world. Everything is correct about that lens; it is an inescapable part of who she is. But let her use that lens how she wants; don't let others tell her how to use it, or to hide it, or to only bring it out when it suits them. It's hers and it's a part of her. I would like her to be proud of that.

—MERIAH NICHOLS

OUR EXPERIENCE: The Search

We started searching about six months before Carter's third birthday. I started with a list of thirteen schools, only five of which offered an integrated setting. Many of the classrooms I saw had children who were nonverbal and at a level, developmentally, that was much lower than where he was currently. Of those [schools], only two would consider Carter for their program. It was clear that one had already decided his placement without meeting my son or even glancing at his evaluations.

I was upset about the limitations that were being put on my son. I received an e-mail from one of our two top choices [saying] that they didn't feel Carter was the right "fit" for their program. I was heartbroken and sure that we would end up at a school that I wasn't happy with and that wouldn't challenge our son. That day, I received a phone call from our top choice. The director said, "We would love to have Carter join our program in the fall. Everyone just fell in love with him. He is the perfect candidate for our school and we'd be honored to have him." Finally. I let out a sigh of relief and joy.

—STACEY CALCANO

OUR EXPERIENCE: The Choice

I was on the homeschooling path and we moved to the Lost Coast of California. The k–12 school here is under 100 kids. It turns out that a man with Down syndrome went through the system and currently plays an integral role with the school. Furthermore, the teacher who would be Moxie's is also a horse therapist and has a background in special education. Yes, this is public school! We enrolled Moxie in the school, of course, and she participates in speech therapy through the school. She engages in horse therapy with her teacher when she is not in school. She also homeschools with me when we travel for six months each year. She has a slice of each life: the more standard public education for half of the year, but in a very rural, intimate setting, and the more radical life with the homeschooling and travel. I believe the two ways are complementary and serve each other well.

—MERIAH NICHOLS

Writing the IEP

When your child reaches the age of three, he or she will be eligible for preschool. The Individual Family Service Plan (IFSP), discussed in Chapter 4, will be a guiding tool as you work with your local school to write an Individualized Education Plan (IEP). We'll discuss IEPs and your child's rights more in Chapter 7. A basic explanation: the IFSP focuses on the child and family and the services that a family needs to help them enhance the development of their child. In contrast, the IEP focuses on the educational needs of the child. Review the following chart for a deeper understanding of the two plans.

FEATURES OF THE INDIVIDUALIZED FAMILY SERVICE PLAN (IFSP) AND THE INDIVIDUALIZED EDUCATION PROGRAM (IEP)	
IFSP	**IEP**
Used in early intervention for children ages birth through 2 and their families	Used in special education for children ages 3 to 21
Includes information about the child's present levels of development	Includes information about the child's present levels of educational performance and participation in developmentally appropriate activities
With the family's approval, it may also include information regarding the family's resources, priorities, and concerns related to the development of their child	Includes information about the family's concerns for enhancing the child's education
After the team determines a list of priorities and concerns, the family determines which outcomes will be included on the IFSP	The IEP team, including the parents or guardians and related service providers who work with the child, determines the goals
Includes the major outcomes desired for the child and family, as well as the methods, timelines, and a plan to measure progress	Includes measurable annual goals, academic and functionality, designed to: Enable the child to be involved in and make progress in the general curriculum; describe how progress will be measured and how often; describe how progress will be reported to the family
Includes the natural environments where services will be provided	Describes services provided in the least restrictive environments (LREs) and an explanation of the extent, if any, that the child will not participate with typically developing children
Includes the early intervention services and supports necessary to meet the unique needs of the child and family in order to achieve the identified outcomes	Includes the special education, related services, supplemental aides and services, modifications, and supports to be provided to help the child make progress and participate in developmentally appropriate activities
Team membership includes: A parent or parents of the child; other family members as requested by the parent; an advocate or person outside the family, if parent requests that the person participate; service coordinator; a person or persons involved in conducting evaluations and assessments	Team membership includes: A parent or parents of the child; regular education teacher; special education teacher; a representative of the school district who can commit resources; a person who can interpret results of the evaluations; others

	who have knowledge or special expertise about the child

Reprinted with permission from PACER Center, Minneapolis, MN, *www.pacer.org*.

The First Day

Now that all the plans are in place, it is time for your child to make his way into the preschool world. Those first days with any child are emotional for any parent, but the added efforts and team planning to make your child with Down syndrome's first be as you envisioned can cause a stir of many feelings.

OUR EXPERIENCE: First Day of School

Nervous, but proud, too. Ben walked right in, sat down with the Play-Doh, and didn't bother to say goodbye to me.

—DEBORAH TOMEI

I bawled my eyes out the day I dropped Everett off for the first time. Now I'm sad to see his preschool end for the summer. He loves it so much; I have to chase him down every day and make him go home with me.

—CARA JACOCKS

Nervous as heck! I think by worrying so much it went that much smoother!

—LAUREN BIEGLER

Excited! Having attended his early intervention play group three days a week, being transported by the van, from age two to age three, by the time preschool came, he was a seasoned professional in both riding the school bus and leaving his mom!

—KAREN GREGOIRE

Proud, relieved, nervous, unsure, happy—all wrapped up in one! And she totally rocked it!

—TRACEY GRAHAM

After all of the meetings, it came down to this day. The day Carsten would wear his backpack, and climb up on that big yellow bus for his first day of preschool. I remember looking down at him as he held my hand to the bus. His smile was huge, and his backpack looked equally huge on his tiny body. Once aboard, his eyes could barely peer out of the bus window to see me. His tiny hand rapidly waved to me. I smiled back at him with one hand waving and the other grabbing my heart because I was certain it was going to fall out right there in the middle of the cul-de-sac. I watched through teary eyes as the bus pulled away with my baby aboard wondering how I would restrain myself from chasing it.

—MEGAN CHISTOFFERSON

Advice from the PT: Motor Skills

"Set high expectations at school and home—expect independence!" says physical therapist Kristi Allison. "Communicate with preschool staff so you know what they are assisting your child with during the day. For example, if the teacher must help take a coat off and hang it on the hook, hang a hook at home and make time to practice. If your child is lagging behind when walking in line or wanting to hold an adult's hand, practice greater speed and independence while out in your community." Don't think that because your child has Ds he can't help out with chores around the house. Such activity can improve his strength and gross and fine motor skills. As well, such activities teach him to plan and execute a job he hasn't previously done. Allison advises, "Encourage him or her to pick up toys, push the full laundry basket, pull clothes out of the dryer, lift dishes out of the dishwasher and hand them overhead to you, or carry light groceries. Start exploring fitness activities such as swimming, biking, or hiking. Demonstrate to your child that being active is important in fostering better health and lifelong fitness."

Advice from the SLP—Speech Development

"Between the ages of three and five your child will start to use many words," says speech-language pathologist Jennifer Bekins. "To continue building your child's vocabulary skills, focus on words that occur frequently throughout her day. These include words associated with routines, like bathing and dressing, toys, and family member names. Next, begin to emphasize descriptive words. For instance, when your child says, 'ball,' model a phrase like, 'Ball. A big ball!' This will help your child understand how to combine words together."

As is true with most babies, your child probably understands far more than she can articulate with her language skills. Keep this in mind when you're speaking to her and about her. Understandably, both you and your child may find this frustrating; she wants to tell you something but doesn't have the words for it. "Support her desire to communicate by offering options when possible," advises Bekins. "For instance, at snack time ask, 'Do you want Goldfish or pretzels?' Provide praise when she answers with speech, signs, or gestures rather than whining."

Keep in mind that your child's speech may be hard to understand. This is where the assistance of a trained speech-language pathologist will be invaluable. Such a professional can work with you to help you communicate successfully with your child. "If therapy is recommended," says Bekins, "it is important for you to be a part of each session. The key to improving your child's communication is to integrate techniques learned from the SLP in your everyday routines."

Advice from the OT—Learning and Practicing Skills

Key activities when your child was younger will change during this period of his life. To review some of the most important:

- **Feeding.** Children with Down syndrome may need to progress from small pieces of food that can be more easily managed. Foods cut into sticks can be used to practice taking bites and facilitate chewing to continue to develop strength and coordination. They are continuing to develop proficiency with utensil use, and they are developing independence with higher-level skills such as opening containers, transferring and pouring food, and helping with food preparation. They have probably outgrown their highchair but still may need support for their best posture.
- **Play.** Play time has become a time for developing muscle strength and gross motor coordination. This is the age where children are further developing their hand skills for prewriting and scissor activities. Use of sensory materials, including touch, movement, and push and pull activities help not only to improve motor skills but also increase your child's attention for higher-level learning.
- **Bath.** Now's the time to work on potty training and dressing skills. Visual supports may help establish the routine: First . . . next . . . all done! Bath time offers the opportunity to sequence and then master a challenging childhood task.

Medical Care/Considerations

Continue to review the AAP guidelines for care of those with Down syndrome at well-child visits and update your care notebook (Chapter 4) as your child grows. Schedule regular checkups to monitor hearing, vision, and dental needs.

Atlantoaxial Instability

In addition to the annual bloodwork and tests your medical team has been reviewing each year, by age three, they will also look at your child's atlantoaxial instability (AI) via the cervical spine. Because people with Down syndrome tend to have loose ligaments and joints, doctors will review your child's neck to determine additional risks or precautions you should consider as your child gets more active. If your child has had surgery, this may have been reviewed before a breathing tube was placed. Having a baseline x-ray of the cervical spine at this age may provide information to guide those decisions. There are varying opinions on when to complete this exam and how much information it truly provides to parents. Talk with your medical team about risks and concerns prior to enrolling in contact sports.

In years past, this test was recommended earlier, but in 2011 the AAP revised its guidelines to begin at age three since bone is more fully formed at that point. They also recommend that if there are concerns revealed by the x-ray, you and your child should be referred to an AI expert in the fields of pediatric orthopedic surgery or pediatric neurosurgery. For more information visit *www.dsmig.org.uk*.

Toilet Training

Few parents look forward to potty training with any child. While most parents are excited to put the diaper years behind them, the thought of the work involved with toilet training can be daunting. A child with Down syndrome may not be fully toilet trained for many years, or he could reach that milestone on target with typical children. It is important to consider your child's needs as you begin the process. Dr. Nancy Grace explains, "I don't use chronological age to determine a child's readiness to begin using the toilet, but feel it's more important that there are a few (very few) signs of readiness." According to Dr. Grace, successful toilet training begins with a child who is able to respond to some minimal degree of instruction and a parent who is willing and able to put effort in the process.

Dr. Grace also provides these keys to success:

- Avoid starting during a phase of change or stress.
- Make the bathroom moderately fun, but not too fun.
- Give the child reinforcements—a small positive reinforcement like a candy or treat. This creates anticipation that the child will get to do something else more fun when he has finished.
- Place children in underwear throughout the process.
- Ensure a child is successful during the day for three to four months before beginning nighttime training.

Ready, Set, Go!

Pre-training (teaching your child to sit cooperatively on the toilet):

1. Have your child sit on the toilet multiple times a day.
2. Start off in small increments (15–30 seconds).
3. Provide low-level engagement—fun, but not *too* fun.
4. Block the child from leaving and redirect if the child wants to leave the room before the time is up.
5. Reward your child for cooperation.

Let the training begin!

1. Give yourself 3–4 days without distraction to get a good head start.
2. Use underwear full-time (exceptions are nighttime and travel time).
3. Schedule sits on the toilet every 30–45 minutes.
4. Prompt communication for using the bathroom (words, sign, whatever works!).
5. Provide lots of fluids.
6. Reward the voiding (and don't be stingy!).

Remain patient and calm during the process. There will probably be accidents and certainly lots of laundry. Collect data on how it is going. Is your child succeeding? Is it time to slow down or speed up? What might be a more effective technique for your child? Reflect as you go and remember: it may take time, but he'll get it!

For more details from Dr. Grace, visit *www.kennedykrieger.org*.

OUR EXPERIENCE: Toilet Training

I was ambitious when we started. Penny was two and a half, and I was convinced that with enough willpower on my part, she could learn to use the potty. I had heard plenty of moms with typically developing children say, 'I just chose a week in the summer and put them in underpants, and by the end of the week we were done.' I knew it might take a little longer, but I figured Penny really wasn't that different from all the other kids. Then came the moment. Penny was sitting on the wooden stairs in my parents' house, and she stood up with a puddle underneath her. I almost burst into tears. And I heard the disappointment in my voice as I said, 'Oh, Penny!' It was then that I knew that this goal was for me, not for her. We put the underwear away for nearly a year.

The funny thing was, even in her Pull-Up, Penny would wander into our room in the middle of the night and say, 'I need to go potty.' And she would. Nearly every night. Last June, we were on a long car trip, and she said, 'I need to go potty.' She held it for twenty minutes as we looked for a place to exit the highway. These moments helped me to realize that in this area, she really is different from other kids. If she's on a playground, with her body and brain focused upon climbing a ladder or hanging from a bar, she doesn't 'hear' the signals that she needs to go. If she's sitting still or sound asleep—if the rest of her body is quiet—then she does. And then there's her low muscle tone, which makes it harder to hold it in even if she knows she needs to. Not to mention the impulsivity that makes her prefer to keep playing, even with wet underwear. I started to understand Penny's hurdles, and I started to respect her more with every try.

So we bought training pants—super absorbent white underwear with strong elastic to prevent further leaking. And we did a lot, a lot, of laundry. We stopped paying attention if she had an accident, and started praising her effusively when she succeeded in going on the potty. For a time, we used M&M's as a reward. Eventually, we got into a rhythm. Every two to two-and-a-half hours, we take a trip to the potty. She's become more and more compliant the more successful she's been. And once it was clear that a day without accidents was a distinct possibility—once it was clear that she could succeed—we introduced 'star' days. After her first star day, we all got ice cream. Then, two in a row, and more chocolate yumminess dripped down her white shirt. Then, three in a row. Four. We don't even talk about star days anymore. But we are working on helping Penny tell us before she needs to go, and we may use stars again once she starts to be able to do so.

Potty training has taken a long time. A really long time. It has set us apart from other families. And it has forced me to listen to Penny. In her own way, she asked me to slow down, to get to know her. She asked me to continue to learn how to love her—not for who I thought I wanted her to be, but acknowledging her needs and her abilities, for who she is. Potty training has been one of the hardest aspects to our life with a child with Down syndrome. It's also been one of the best.

—AMY JULIA BECKER, AUTHOR OF *A GOOD AND PERFECT GIFT*. ESSAY PUBLISHED ORIGINALLY AT *HTTP://BLOOM-PARENTINGKIDSWITHDISABILITIES.BLOGSPOT.COM*.

Extra-Curricular Activities

Fostering independence and friendships is important for anyone, including children with Down syndrome. Today there are lots of options available for activities—ones that are inclusive and ones that are geared toward children with disabilities. Contact your local Down syndrome groups, school, and city recreation office for a list of activities to consider.

OUR EXPERIENCE: Local Recreation Leagues

Brianne is five and has Down syndrome. Her brother is four. We signed them both up for a soccer league and loved having them on the same team. I was a bit hesitant as I worried how she would do on a "typical" team . . . but I assured myself since it's youth soccer, it would be fine. It was more than fine—it was fabulous! Watching three- to five-year-olds play soccer is some of the best entertainment ever. Kiddos running in all directions —boys stopping to look at ladybugs, girls twirling in circles until they are dizzy, and a few soccer stars who have serious skills. The first few games Brianne didn't spend much time on the field since she would wander off for a drink break or to sit on the sidelines, but by the end of the season she was lasting for most or all of her time . . . although sometimes she would get distracted and spin herself so dizzy she'd fall down or sit in the goal and play with the net—but other kiddos were having these same distractions, so it was perfectly fine. We were very impressed with how the team and coaches included Brianne and treated her just like any other teammate.

—ADRIENNE SULLIVAN

Special Olympics

Since 1968, the Special Olympics has offered athletes with intellectual disabilities a place to learn, play, and grow. Their mission is to serve children and adults with intellectual disabilities through year-round sports training and competitions, to provide many Olympic-style sports and aim to "develop physical fitness, demonstrate courage, experience joy, and participate in a sharing of gifts, skills, and friendship with their families, other Special Olympics athletes, and the community."

The Special Olympics Young Athlete Program (YAP) serves children ages two to seven with a focus on games and activities that promote fun and further development of motor skills and hand/eye coordination. The YAP is one that is intended to be inclusive, welcoming children with and without disabilities to participate. To join, or to get a program started, visit *www.specialolympics.org/young_athletes* for more information.

OUR EXPERIENCE: Special Olympics

I started Greyson (two) in the Young Athletes Program even before he could walk because I wanted him to grow up believing in himself that he could do anything he set his mind to. Each week, Greyson is learning to overcome his disabilities amongst his peers, who also have a wide variety of disabilities. We celebrate the achievements no matter how small. His sibling, Addison (three), joins him weekly and she is learning very young that everyone is an individual and that people of all ages are not labeled by their disability.

—KELLY FRENCH

OUR EXPERIENCE: The Preschool Years

Nico's transition to preschool was pretty great, at first. He went from days of therapy at home to half days in a classroom with five to eight other children all with varying special needs. It was a good transition from home, but it wasn't until we moved and switched districts that we realized it was no longer the best fit for Nico. He was missing the social interaction that would support his independence and learning. We were a bit nervous making the switch; the classrooms were vastly different. Nico went from a small, fully contained early childhood class to an inclusive classroom comprised of students with and without disabilities. Yet in the new school we saw our son flourish and thrive. With the increased social interaction, he was growing as a student and person, and this was exciting to see. As I look back on that time, a critical part of the school transition we learned was to regularly re-evaluate placement for our son. In our case, it happened due to the move, but it caused us to intentionally reflect more often about the environment and how well it was meeting his needs. As parents, we need to ask ourselves, "Is this the correct environment for our child?" That reflection allows us to better plan for next steps and create the right educational setting for our students.

—DAVID PERRY

At three, Bobby still had a lot of medical needs due to his heart condition. He had a feeding tube, could not walk, etc. We chose a self-contained school (100 percent special needs) with a full-time nursing staff. Safety was our first priority. Second was the fact it was an all-day program with full-time therapists and a four-to-one student/teacher ratio—he had so many delays we wanted him to have extra opportunities to grow. We kept him there for three years while he got healthy and subsequently took off developmentally. This year he started kindergarten at a neighborhood school and has done great. He just needed that extra support in the beginning.

—ANNE GRUNSTED

There is a mountain to climb therapeutically for children with Down syndrome. As a parent navigating this mountain, it is overwhelming at times between physical, occupational, cognitive, and speech therapies. We were fortunate enough to have a pediatrician who also had a child with Down syndrome. She's been a constant resource for us regarding the latest research and best therapies. In the beginning, she helped us prioritize our son's therapies on speech and comprehension. While we knew all therapies for him were important, we really doubled down on these two therapies. The theory was that if our child was to get ahead in these areas, then his world would open up in the best ways possible. With her advice, and our own research, we introduced a reading program called Love and

Learning and the Signing Times DVDs to our son at the age of one. We want to be clear that neither of these programs felt overwhelming and easily fit into our life schedules. We strongly believe this early engagement had profound effects on his cognition levels and his speaking clarity. Our son is now six and can read somewhere around a second-grade level. As for his speech, many therapists note his high level of articulation. We aren't sure this would be the case if we did not get such great advice early from our pediatrician and other resources in the Ds community.

—ROB AND ELLEN SNOW

Resources

For Your Information

- Parent Resource Center: *www.parentcenterhub.org/resources*
- Milestone Information: *www.dsmig.org.uk*
- IDSC groups for preschool-adult children: *http://theidsc.org/resources*

Chapter Seven
Primary and Middle School

The next phase of your child's life includes teaching students and educators, individuals and the community, parents and children. This age is when you make your initial school decisions, choose and balance educational priorities, develop and tune IEPS, and throughout it all teach and encourage positive social interactions.

> **Dear New Parents,**
> Perhaps you've heard that special-needs children and their parents need to battle with the schools and the system. The reason you may battle is simple—you now see your child for the complex bundle of potential that she is. You know she's great at (fill in the blank) even if she's not great at (fill in the blank), and you will not let anyone box her into a set of limitations.

School Choices & Priorities

Here are things to consider when you're choosing a school: Academic reputation, inclusion standards/priority within the typical classroom, transportation considerations, school policies in regard to safety and discipline, homework rules and expectations, student rights and responsibilities, whole child education (art, therapies, recess, music, etc.), and financial requirements. First and foremost consider your child's strengths, weaknesses, and unique abilities for making the best possible matchup, as you would with any of your children.

Introduce Your Child

Help the typical peers of your child by visiting your child's class personally. Read a story and talk about your child, how he or she is like the other children and also mention the differences. Provide the tools to make inclusion work. For example, the book *My Name Is Sean and I Have Something to Share* by Sandra Assimotos McElwee includes both conversation prompts for the children as well as a "letter to the parents" template.

Public School

The most common choice for parents is the public school system. Often, a child with special needs has already attended a public preschool with an individualized education plan (IEP) plan in place. This is a great advantage, as the transition from preschool to elementary school is in process. At this point in a child's life, families already experience the benefits of the legal responsibilities required of the public school system mandated by the Individuals with Disabilities Education Act (IDEA), which incorporates a Free Appropriate Public Education (FAPE) individualized for each student.

Education-Related Acronyms

As you journey through this new world full of acronyms, here's a quick guide to what these letters represent.

- **IDEA:** Originally "The Education of All Handicapped Children Act," which passed in 1970 and was renamed the Individuals with Disabilities Education Act (IDEA). Because of this act, children with disabilities receive education via the public schools; it has been revised several times, most recently in 2004.
- **FAPE:** Part of the IDEA, this stands for Free Appropriate Public Education.
- **NCLB:** No Child Left Behind Act, designed to hold schools accountable and improve student achievement levels.
- **IEP:** Individualized Education Program. The plan for a student's goal achievement assembled in cooperation with the teachers, specialists, other interested parties, the student, and the family.
- **HEOA:** The Higher Education Opportunity Act, enacted in 2008, reauthorizing the Higher Education Act (HEA) of 1965. This law contains a number of important new provisions that improve access to post-secondary education for students with intellectual disabilities.

Be sure to include the goals of your child and which school is best equipped to handle these goals in the IEP process. If you disagree with the placement your district recommends for your child, you may have to familiarize yourself (and the school) with your child's legal rights. If it comes to this, Wrightslaw.com has resources to help you get started.

Private School

Families that prioritize a faith-based private school for their child can often find a program. Sometimes a public school system will enable specialists, e.g., a speech or occupational therapist, to meet a student with special needs at a private school in order to fill in these areas. In some cases a public school system has paid a private school when the public school cannot meet a child's needs, however this is unusual, and if you choose a private school the cost will most likely be your responsibility.

You may also have to pay if additional therapists are needed for your child, so it is a good idea to check the public school system's policies before you commit yourself.

Some areas have faith-based schools that are specialized for the education of developmentally delayed students. That's the case with Jayne, Lane's mom, who says, "In two years, a few big accomplishments academically are: writing his first and last name, trying to read, and copying words from the board or from other papers. Lane enjoys learning and loves to go to the Madonna School."

Note that while private schools are, technically, not required by law to adhere to the IDEA rules and regulations, or enforce an IEP program, you should consider how they implement these or similar rules as part of their curriculum for serving a student with Down syndrome.

Homeschool

Many families across the country choose to homeschool their children, whether differently abled or not. Each state has specific regulations regarding homeschooling, testing, curriculum, and process.

If you homeschool, you may engage specialists to cover particular needs of your child. In some places a homeschool and public school cooperative option allows a student to go to the school for specialized needs, while the family homeschools for the balance of academics. This option has to be specially arranged and often still requires/involves an IEP with the public school team.

Choosing Top Priorities

When looking at school alternatives, consider these three steps:

1. Choose the *top* priorities and the *top* deal breakers. For example, is inclusion the most important value? Or is it academics?
2. Research and visit the school. Communicate with the school *before* your student is enrolled. Also, check the statistics, teacher turnover, and go "old-school" by asking around.
3. Adjust as needed. Keep in mind that the best learning environment for your child at age six may not be the same at age ten.

Resources

- *My Name Is Sean and I Have Something to Share* by Sandra Assimotos McElwee
- Laws by State Regarding Homeschooling: *www.hslda.org/laws*

Introduction to the IEP

IEP was borne of federal legislation (IDEA) to enable children with disabilities to get a free, appropriate, public education. The IEP meeting and plan is put together by the team of professionals and interested parties that are involved in the education of the student. According to the U.S. Department of Education, the public agency must ensure that the IEP team for each child with a disability includes:

- The parents
- At least one regular education teacher of the child (if the child is, or may be, participating in the regular education environment)
- At least one special education teacher
- A representative of the school district
- Someone who can interpret the child's test results
- Anyone else who has special knowledge or expertise regarding the child
- Finally, where it's appropriate, the child

Most often the IEP team meets where the services are performed and meets once a year, but the plan can be revised and updated between official meetings.

Why an IEP?

1. **For the student.** The system continues to evolve and improve to provide an education that will enable and empower your child to learn academics, as well as give her the independence, self-esteem, and satisfaction that comes from learning.
2. **For the professionals.** By working with the parents to establish goals, taking the time to analyze your child's specific needs, and others who are experienced with the specialties that educating your child may entail.

3. **For you.** The knowledge that steps are taken on a daily basis to give your son or daughter the public education that will take him or her to the next phase of academics and independence.

How Does the Process Work?

Every IEP meeting will discuss the following issues:

- Your child's present levels of academic achievement and functional performance
- Annual goals
- How the progress will be measured
- The special education, related services, and supplementary aids and services that will be provided to (or on behalf of) your child, including program modifications or supports for school staff
- An explanation of the extent (if any) to which your child will or will not participate with children without disabilities
- Any modifications your child will need when taking statewide or district-wide assessments
- The dates when services will begin and end, the amount of services, as well as how often and where they will take place
- How and when you will be informed of your child's progress

IEP Team

The IEP team is created to give your student the tools she needs to succeed. No one team member can (or should) be all things to your child's education. Work to develop your child's unique strengths first, and follow with the request for accommodations as needed.

Write everything down to help everyone be clear on decisions and responsibilities. The teachers and school administrators have many parents to meet, so your IEP meeting may be between other parent meetings. If time runs short, request another meeting.

For additional support, contact your local DSA; they will guide you to other parents and resources specific to your area. Check your school district website for specific information about special education and the IEP process; its guidelines and tips will let you know what to expect from their placed procedures.

Above all, communicate with your team about your child's strengths and ambitions. As an example, here is a letter written by Amy Dietrich Hernandez to her son's IEP team as he transitioned into high school.

Dear Team,

This is my son, Charles. We are here to find the best possible placement for him. Before we do that, however, I want to remind you that he is not just a set of strengths and weaknesses. He is a teenager, a much-loved son and brother, a good friend, and a bundle of wit and sarcasm. He wants what all of us want out of life: to love and be loved, to have friends and to be included. That last part is tricky, because it can't really be quantified. I am afraid that sometimes, the human being gets lost in the graphs and percentiles. I am afraid that for some, my Charles is a challenge at best and a problem at worst.

Inclusion is not a pie-in-the-sky fantasy; it is the only way to ensure that my child's life is seen as having as much value as those of his typical peers. If you think I am exaggerating, consider what happens when people are segregated from society. Times have changed for people with Down syndrome, but until stories of prom kings and queens and team managers are more than feel-good anecdotes, people like my son will not be fully participating members of society, and that is what I want for my son. My husband and I want full participation in life (not just school) for Charles and every child who comes after him.

I look forward to the day Charles walks across the stage in his cap and gown, ready to accept his certificate and to step into a world that is more accepting and inclusive than it is today, because of the work of teams like this.

Thank you.

[Charles's parents]

Resources

- IDEA: *http://idea.ed.gov*
- WrightsLaw: *www.wrightslaw.com*
- Parent Center Hub: *www.parentcenterhub.org/repository/pa12*
- *IEP and Inclusion Tips for Parents and Teachers* by Anne Eason and Kathleen Whitbread: *www.attainmentcompany.com/iep-and-inclusion-tips-parents-and-teachers*

Developing Social Skills

Social skills include everything your child needs to participate successfully in environments like school or work, concepts like turn-taking, how to hold a conversation, and problem solving. Most importantly, demonstrating social skills is the first step to your child effectively advocating for himself. Consequently, teaching a solid base of appropriate social skills and communication, with the understanding and guidance of you and your child's teachers, empowers him to thrive as a self-advocate and active member of his community.

Some of the more common challenges faced by a child with Ds include: sensory sensitivities, inclination to "wander," communication barriers, and/or a dual diagnosis such as autism, anxiety, or attention deficit disorder. All of these challenges require additional planning, education, and habit creation. Doing so helps your child to manage and eventually thrive in social situations. Involve teachers, grandparents, siblings, and even neighbors in the education and implementation of planning and reacting to these areas of a child's social stimulation.

Stereotypes

"All children with Down syndrome are *so* friendly." "*They all* love people so much." "They all . . ." Although often well intentioned, these stereotypes not only reduce people with Down syndrome to a caricature, but also, ironically, add pressure via expectation to act or be a certain way. Every child is born with his/her own unique personality. Teaching social skills is one way we, as parents, help our child to be true to herself.

Don't ignore "stubbornness." Children learn when they are held accountable in social situations. Stubbornness can even be an important health cue. Is a young child stubborn, or in fact is he having difficulty hearing? Or are there troubles with a child's sleep patterns, causing her to have difficulty concentrating? As parents, we must watch the cues our children give while not making assumptive jumps based on stereotypes.

Safety

Sometimes empowering our children means we have to talk to them about boundaries, bullying, and even running from danger. KidPower.org is a website that has many resources on teaching safety to children of all abilities, including webinars, articles, and for-sale comic books.

Inclusion Begins at Home

Community events and inclusion with typical peers is one part of the process to help any child, both by watching and interacting. Children (and adults) should be enrolled and encouraged in school and community age-appropriate events when possible. Expect the best from the community. Inclusion is a great teacher of a child with Ds, and also a great teacher of acceptance.

Most local Down syndrome organizations have a calendar full of events to choose from. The Arc is a great organizer of family activities, and also check out regional camps that understand and embrace the unique strengths and abilities of children with Down syndrome. Another event that builds self-esteem and encourages the positive muscle work of action and activity is the Special Olympics. As with most skills, parents and educators encourage and reinforce a child's behavior, but the true learning comes from peer interaction.

Resources

- Kidpower Safety Comics Series: *www.kidpower.org/store/safety-comics*
- Special Olympics: *www.specialolympics.org*

Chapter Eight
Teenage Years

In 1989, television introduced a character with Down syndrome into homes around the world. *Life Goes On* featured actor Chris Burke as Corky and showed life for a teenager with Down syndrome and his family. The first season's plots revolved almost exclusively around Corky, his school, and challenges, but as the show evolved the focus broadened to wider issues and characters. This is similar to real life. When a child with Down syndrome is born, the world seems to revolve around "Down syndrome" for a while, until . . . it doesn't anymore. By the time your child with Down syndrome becomes a teenager, you have long since recognized the unique strengths, attributes, and personality of your child. Metaphorically, the camera pans out to the wider view as your family lives your day-to-day lives.

Dear New Parents,

Almost the moment a student enters high school, the planning begins to transition your child into adult life. While other parents are encouraging their kids to "Be a kid—you only live once!" educators start telling you to "Plan! Plan! Plan!" It's intimidating. Even more intimidating is that the transition from teenage years to adulthood is called *The Cliff*, by both agencies and families within the disability community. The good news? Life goes on. Ready or not, tomorrow comes. So it begins, the big transition: graduation and choosing post-secondary school options, including college.

High School Social Skills

As a person with Ds reaches high school, staying social and learning the skills needed to build and hold relationships with educators, bosses, and peers continues to elevate in importance. As mentioned in the previous chapter, appropriate social skills ultimately enable a person to hold a job, have friends, enjoy self-confidence, and develop a network of support.

What Makes Friendship

In children, simple proximity is perhaps the biggest factor in building friendships. Why are two kids friends? Because they live next door and can play together every day. In some ways, this continues into adulthood; how many friends have you made at work? Similar interests is another factor that people build relationships upon, leading to thousands of complete strangers being "friends" for one day when their favorite sports team plays. Then, as friendships mature, the elements of loyalty, reliance on one another, and companionship evolve.

The reason these factors are important to consider as parents and educators of people with disabilities is that it is up to us to facilitate circumstances where friendship can blossom. For example, a person can't make friends if he never leaves the house. A person can't make friends if she isn't allowed to explore things of interest to her, preferably in a group, so that she can connect with others who have that same interest.

Challenges

There are certain challenges faced by some people with Ds that need to be considered when promoting and teaching in social environments.

As mentioned previously, some people with Ds may also have sensory sensitivities and/or a dual diagnosis such as autism, anxiety, or ADD. These people need to work with specialists and have to make an extra effort to succeed in social situations within the limitations these conditions may impose. As a child progresses, there will be new adventures and challenges to work within or overcome. Speech and language delays probably cause the greatest challenge for creating relationships and pursuing social interactions.

Professor Sue Buckley, OBE, Director of Science and Research, Down Syndrome Education International, observes, "The social and emotional effects of limited spoken language abilities become more significant during this life stage, and will affect the quality of life of adults with Down syndrome if they are not addressed."

Consequently, you, as well as your child's teachers, must keep language and communication skills as a top priority throughout your student's career. It is, unfortunately, not unusual for schools to drop speech as a priority as a student ages. Keep in mind, your child will continue to learn and grow as long as she is given the opportunity and tools to do so.

Social skills are learned actions, reactions, and behaviors. As the person with Down syndrome reaches middle and high school years, consider checking the local DSA or The Arc for classes for teens with intellectual and developmental disabilities (I/DD). They often offer special sessions on subjects such as dating, making friends, and even looking your best. Role-playing with peers can be the best learning environment.

Learning from Doing

Just as when children are young, there are a variety of social opportunities within the Down syndrome and I/DD community that promote lifelong friendships and positive social interaction with peers.

In fact, throughout the lifespan of a person with Ds, the Special Olympics offers activities promoting sportsmanship and positive interactions. Best Buddies International begins their programming at the middle school grade level. This is a particularly important time for learning socialization, and the one-on-one partnerships and mentoring enable the child to build self-confidence and learn social cues that are so important for later self-advocacy.

Another program that matches people with Down syndrome with a typical peer is Camp PALS. The camp experience is offered to teens and young adults at camps around the country. Their website, PalsPrograms.org, says, "PALS Programs provides a place for young adults with Down syndrome and their peers to have fun, grow as individuals, and build transformative friendships."

In School and in the Community

In high school, parents often see greater changes, limitations, and struggles regarding school inclusion. Consequently, it is important that your child have social skills and interaction with typical peers as part of the IEP process in order to garner support from the school system. If possible, recruit and reinforce the teacher's role in encouraging positive social behaviors and even enable meaningful cooperation and companionship. Building friendships can be part of the IEP, as this is one of the most important "life skills" that a person can have. The booklet *IEP and Inclusion Tips for Parents and Teachers* by Anne Eason and Kathleen Whitbread reminds parents to watch for situations that are barriers to making friends, like too many hovering adults, or similarly too little access to peers. Communicate with the school officials and ask, "Who is friendly and has similar strengths and interests?" and "Can you arrange a meaningful social or educational activity so my child can hang out with other students?" Promote areas that create positive social interaction experiences.

OUR EXPERIENCE: Rachel and Student Council

At the beginning of the school year, Rachel ran for student council. We worked on posters. She did her little speech. She handed out candy. Election day came.

"Guess what, Mom. I was elected as a member at large!" She was thrilled.

The student council vice president is an amazing young woman, too. (She is headed off to become a special education teacher and will be an amazing one.) She has started calling Rachel from time to time and inviting her to do things. Rachel getting a phone call from a senior she idolizes does make her feel pretty important. That wouldn't have happened if she hadn't taken that chance and gotten involved.

She has loved being a part of student council (STUCO). Really that goes to the point of it all. We all want to be a part of something. We all want to belong—remember Maslow's Hierarchy of Needs, anyone? Rachel is no different.

Rachel got the "Best School Spirit" award for "being so optimistic and happy all the time! We couldn't do it without you." Once again, she was thrilled, you would think she had won an Oscar!

And now about that inclusion thing . . . Who does benefit from inclusion? I think the answer is pretty clear.

—ORIGINALLY PUBLISHED BY JAWANDA MAST ON THESASSYSOUTHERNGAL.COM. REPRINTED BY PERMISSION.

Note to Parents on Bullies

According to PACER's National Bullying Prevention Center, studies have recently "proven" what many parents have always known: People with disabilities are more likely to be bullied. If your child is being bullied at school, this is a violation of his civil rights and needs to be brought to the school administrator's attention. Over the past few years the FAPE, Free and Public Education laws, include the clarification that bullying in the school interferes with education and is therefore the responsibility of the school officials to prevent and stop.

Community

Once a student reaches middle school and beyond, it is likely their interests begin to blossom. Expand these areas with social activities within the community. As mentioned previously, get your child with like-minded peers, whether it is comic books, drama, or sports. Most of all, recognize that each person is unique and play to her or his social strengths and interests.

OUR EXPERIENCE: Rion at Camp

Years ago, we went to a Christian camp for a week. Students begin the week signing up for activities in which they would like to participate. Rion signed up for water sports. After a few games of beach-ball volleyball, they divided the teens up for a relay race, four kids per team. I watched as Rion's three teammates saw him assigned to their team. Now maybe I should mention . . . Rion was the only child at camp with a disability. It was clear these kids figured they were going to lose. You could see the resigned looks on their faces.

They lined up, Rion bringing up the rear as the fourth man in the relay. What these teens did *not* know is that Rion is a serious competitive swimmer with Special Olympics. Plus, he has participated in the community pool's summer swim league with "typical peers."

Rion's specialty? The butterfly!

Needless to say, his team "smoked" the others. Rion glided across that pool like he was in a swim meet. Through sports, Rion has won the respect of his "typical" peers, but he is also a friendly, accepting person. He loves people, but he gives them space. He doesn't "attach" himself to people making it awkward for others. He knows when to speak, and when to walk away.

As an educator, I have seen many parents of children with special needs asking for accommodations and modifications to make a child's adjustment easier. We never did this. While accommodations are necessary for some children, we felt like the world will not make adjustments for him so it would be better for him to learn how to overcome obstacles without asking for special treatment. We have kept Rion very busy. He participates in church activities, sports, and social events with both his special education peers and his "reg ed" peers. He is a well-rounded young man now with friends galore!

—ORIGINALLY PUBLISHED BY SUSAN HOLCOMBE ON *THE ROAD WE'VE SHARED*

Resources

- PALS Programs: *www.palsprograms.org*
- Best Buddies: *www.bestbuddies.org*
- Special Olympics: *www.specialolympics.org*
- PACER's National Bullying Prevention Center: *www.pacer.org/bullying/resources/students-with-disabilities*
- StopBullying.gov: *www.stopbullying.gov/at-risk/groups/special-needs*
- Speech and Language Development for Teenagers with Down Syndrome (11–16 Years): *http://store.dseusa.org/products/speech-language-development-teenagers-down-syndrome-11-16-years*
- *IEP and Inclusion Tips for Parents and Teachers* by Anne Eason and Kathleen Whitbread: *www.attainmentcompany.com/iep-and-inclusion-tips-parents-and-teachers*

Graduation and Transition

Significant change happens several times throughout a child's school career, from early intervention into primary school, then to middle and high school and sometimes even transitions to new programs. However, transition, *The Big Transition* for which parents, students, and educators take years to prepare, is the transition from school-age into adult living. You will start hearing the term "transition" when it comes to preparing your child for aging out of the school system.

It's not unusual to feel, "There's time . . . there's time . . ." Then suddenly there's an avalanche of things to do! This feeling is why the IDEA requires transition planning to begin by the time your child is sixteen. Some schools choose to include transition planning in the IEPs even earlier.

Because the IDEA includes the option of continuing education for students with learning disabilities until the age of twenty-one, the transition plan includes graduation choices, college or ongoing education plans, vocational training requirements, and attaining social and life skills as well as independent living goals. The transition plan also means you should begin making a checklist of applications and paperwork that may be beneficial to your child as he moves into adulthood. In short, this is going to be a very complicated change, one that requires extensive and cooperative preparation.

Paper Trail

Some of the paperwork you'll begin while your offspring is still in high school includes:

- Acquire a state ID and Social Security card
- Register for selective services
- Begin the application process for SSI and possibly Medicaid

As well, you'll need to:

- Familiarize yourself with the state's rules on guardianship, power of attorney, and so on (more on this in Chapter 9)

- Begin evaluating the need and applications for disability-related benefits with the state
- Begin to evaluate the need for disability-related benefits and Medicaid versus competitive employment and employer insurance

Circle of Support

As the student with Down syndrome reaches an age where she is learning to advocate for herself, this is also a good time to begin developing a "Circle of Support." According to the Foundation for People with Learning Disabilities, "A Circle of Support is a group of people who meet regularly to help someone achieve their ambitions in life." This is an informal group who are involved with, care about, and can advocate for and with the person with Ds.

This circle will surely change over the years. To begin with, the core of the traditional team built and required by IDEA, including peers, family, and friends, will be on this team. As you and your offspring develop a longer-term person-centered plan, you'll add people to the team who empower your son's or daughter's strengths and ambitions.

> **Note to Parents**
>
> Let's face it, our kids sometimes tell their friends or grandparents, or frankly, *anyone but us*, what they are really feeling or thinking about the plan we, as parents, put into place. Make sure your child's Circle of Support includes the people he/she really talks to—the people who "get it."

As your child learns to speak up and self-advocate, this team will continue to work together to empower and partner with her to create the future she wants.

Making a Transition Plan with the School

The first component of the IEP transition plan is to decide when and if the student will graduate with a completion certificate, with the academic requirements for a diploma, or with a GED. Although different states (and even districts within them) have variable options regarding graduation requirements, in most cases if a student is included in the public schools with *any* modifications to the general education, the student's classes do not count as "credit" and will not apply to a standard diploma.

Keep in mind that if your student is learning well with the modified classroom experience and a graduation equivalent is important to his post–high school goals, then preparing for a GED may be an appropriate goal within the IEP. As a college experience becomes increasingly available to teens with learning disabilities, don't cross college off the list of possibilities.

Diploma Options

The National Center on Educational Outcomes says, "Many kinds of diplomas and certificates are used across the U.S. to document that a student has completed school. Some of these diplomas and certificates are just for students receiving special education services. Few states have only the standard diploma available to students. Some states have tests that students must pass to earn a diploma, while others do not."

Every state and even individual school districts have specified information about graduation diplomas and requirements. Ask early to be sure you are on track for the goals of your child.

ADVANTAGES AND DISADVANTAGES OF FOUR DIPLOMA OPTIONS		
Diploma Option/Policy	**Advantages**	**Disadvantages**
Standard Diploma or Better; Single Criteria. A standard diploma or a more rigorous option (e.g., honors diploma) is available to all students. All must meet the same criteria for earning the diploma.	Provides students the "key" to entry into post-secondary institutions or employment. Meaning of earning a	Does not recognize the different learning styles of students with disabilities. May result in a significant number of students not

	diploma is clear because there is only one set of criteria. Maintains high expectations and a focus on the general education curriculum.	receiving any kind of exit document from high school.
Standard Diploma or Better; Multiple Criteria. Some students are allowed to meet one or more of the requirements in different ways from other students (e.g., different courses, meeting IEP goals, exemption).	Recognizes that students have different learning styles and skills that may not align with typical graduation criteria. Ensures that more students will get a diploma than would with a single set of criteria.	Reduces quality control on the knowledge and skills of students leaving school. Results in non-standard sets of knowledge and skills among students, all of whom have the same diploma.
Certificate Options. Certificates for attendance, completion, achievement, etc., are available to all students. Requirements can vary considerably, and may or may not allow students with IEPs to meet them in different ways.	Maintains the integrity of the requirements for earning a standard diploma. Provides other exit options for students not meeting the requirements for a standard diploma.	Produces students with diploma options about which we have little knowledge of their consequences for post-secondary schooling or employment. Flags those students receiving special education services.
Special Education Diploma. Diploma or certificate available only to students with IEPs. This type of diploma typically is added to other options for non-IEP students.	Recognizes that students with disabilities may be working on different standards from other students.	Does not promote access to the general education curriculum.

Chart courtesy of M. Thurlow and S. Thompson, *Diploma Options and Graduation Policies for Students with Disabilities* (Policy Directions No. 10). Minneapolis, MN: University of Minnesota, National Center on Educational Outcomes. *Retrieved 5/31/15, from the World Wide Web:http://education.umn.edu/NCEO/OnlinePubs/Policy10.htm*

The IDEA and Transition

Transition includes a variety of steps, education, and teamwork, and like every other phase of the IDEA implementation must focus on measurable objectives. Because the IDEA is individualized, the law indicates that when it comes to transition planning, begin with your child's long-term goals in mind. Not only are academics to be considered when implementing the education of your child, but also vocational skills, independent living preparation, and community involvement. The transition plan considers post secondary education, job support, and day services as appropriate for your soon-to-be adult son or daughter. The IDEA law mandates that your child's transition plan include:

- Instruction
- Related services
- Community experiences
- The development of employment and other post-school adult living objectives
- If appropriate, acquisition of daily-living skills and provision of a functional vocational evaluation

Transition Programs

Most students with Down syndrome choose to continue with the public schools in what is usually termed a transition program until the age of twenty-one. The transition programs often teach primarily vocational and life skills and focus on preparing the student for post-school life.

Some schools choose to work with specialized vocational programs such as Project SEARCH, which helps young adults with learning disabilities acquire internships and consequent community employment. (Employment options are discussed more thoroughly in the next chapter.)

Transition programs also focus on life skills in the curriculum. Life skills include a variety of tasks and functional concepts, including, but not limited to:

- **Safety and Way Finding**, from crossing the street to learning to use public transportation independently
- **Money Management**, from understanding and counting coins to checking/savings bank phone apps
- **Home living**, from making a bed to safe cooking skills
- **Self-care**, from hand-washing skills to making healthy food choices
- **Others**, including, but not limited to, shopping, Internet use and safety, cleaning, and decision-making

Your family and the teachers you work with need to continually evaluate your student's skills and goals to decide which of these lessons should and can be incorporated into the education plan. What other resources does the child have for learning these skills? For example, if your family has the time and resources to offer your child one-on-one time to facilitate these lessons at home, there may not be a need for the school environment to focus on some of these skills. The IEP should play to your child's strengths as well as incorporate key factors that lead to a life goal.

For example, public transportation has an array of safety and social concerns for parents. However, in many instances it's a person's ticket to work and a more independent adult life. Your son or daughter needs to know how to use it. This is a skill set that will take them time and practice to master. Here's a clear case where your family can help teach the necessary skills.

The school day has a limited number of hours, so your family will have to balance against your own time resources what is the best long-term choice for your child.

Preparing for the transition to post–high school life means checking out all of the options, discussing the wants and strengths of your offspring, and sometimes getting creative with the IEP team to reach the student's goals.

OUR EXPERIENCE: Connor's Evolving Transition Plans

When we started the transition IEPs [when Connor was] fourteen, they (the school team) wanted to shift him into a "life skills" focused format. We said, "No. You're going to test him along with the other kids, even though that will be harder and not necessarily the 'program.'" Which they did and it was.

When we started the transition planning we thought he'd finish high school and we'd look into community college and think part-time jobs. Academically he whizzed through everything to meet his general-ed requirements—well, maybe not whizzed through. That sounds like it was easy and all-accessible for him, curriculum-wise. It was hard for him, and us, with many long evenings of difficult homework on even modified work.

A number of his friends who did not pursue the general track for a variety of reasons are every bit as outgoing, engaged, and engaging young adults now, so it almost seems like it doesn't matter; it all works out. That said, it needs to be a family decision made in the best interests of the individual child, not by and for the convenience of [the] school system looking to plop the kid into a one-size-fits-all existing program that does not really recognize and adapt to the individual strengths, challenges, and needs of the student. Anyway, at seventeen we felt like he needed more maturity; we couldn't see him going into a post-secondary environment (yet). So we said, let's do transition. He's gained a lot from this work experience.

Then when Connor was seventeen, a casting call came up for the film *Menschen* and sparked his interest. Connor costarred in this independent film and began taking acting classes, Shakespearean and all, and re-engaged himself into community theater.

When the acting thing came up at this new level of interest and intensity, we thought, we'll put off a serious look at college right now. You can always do that. At the same time, it was convenient, because (after high school) he just needed more maturity. We didn't feel (in our area) there is the level of support that he would need to go into a community college, because you're too on your own. The logistics would be challenging. So it's worked out. He's more mature now; he's getting new skill sets and developing confidence.

My observation in terms of social interactions (for Connor) is [that] work relationships are fun because of the team atmosphere, and also they are more organic and honest (than school).

—BRIAN LONG

Worry versus Planning

"Plans are nothing; planning is everything," Dwight D. Eisenhower is supposed to have said. In fact, what parents really need to remember is: "Worry is nothing; planning is everything." Instead of wasting energy on worrying about the future, take steps with your child to stand in the center of a solid transition plan. Then be open to change.

Resources

- Recommended Reading: "Higher Expectations to Better Outcomes for Children with Disabilities" via *Homeroom*, the official blog of the U.S. Department of Education:

www.ed.gov/blog/2014/06/higher-expectations-to-better-outcomes-for-children-with-disabilities

- Building a Circle of Support: *www.learningdisabilities.org.uk/help-information/information-for-teachers/transition-to-adulthood/building-circles-of-support*
- Person-Centered Planning: *www.learningdisabilities.org.uk/help-information/information- for-teachers/transition-to-adulthood/using-person-centred- planning*
- IDEA: *http://idea.ed.gov/explore/home*, *http://idea.ed.gov*
- Transition Coalition: *http://transitioncoalition.org*

College and Post-Secondary Education

Although there are not yet validated statistics on how many adults with Down syndrome have attended or are attending college, this does not discount the fact that there are students with Down syndrome both in college programs now and who have attended college programs both with assistance and independently. Currently there are several options available for students with disabilities. Interested students should check with their local college and university's admissions office for information and accommodations for students with special needs.

NOTE FROM THE AUTHOR: SERIOUSLY, COLLEGE!

I love that the options for continuing education are acknowledged and accepted for our adult children with Down syndrome. My son took a class at our local community college and is looking into taking more in the future. In fact, we're thinking of taking a class or two together. The Think College website, at

ThinkCollege.net, currently lists 240 college programs across the country for individuals with developmental disabilities. I expect that's not even all of them, as the community college Marcus enrolled in, with the help of a special coordinator in the college admissions office, is not listed on their website. So, ask whatever college your son or daughter is interested in pursuing and there may be opportunities for enrollment. And that's *today*, as I write this. By the time you're reading this book, there will be more, and when you're researching colleges with your child, it'll be more still.

—Mardra

Two examples of programs specializing in the college experience for young adults with developmental disabilities are ClemsonLIFE and the University of Cincinnati Transition and Access Program. There are currently hundreds of college options to inspire and investigate. Here we'll look at these two examples.

- **ClemsonLIFE:** Features the option of a two- or three-year program that includes functional academics, for example teaching the skills necessary for independent living, including areas like personal banking, filling out job applications, and the social skills required for a successful interview. The students live on campus with a focus on "Interaction with Clemson University students from all across campus." More information at *www.clemson.edu/hehd/departments/education/culife*.
- **The University of Cincinnati:** According to the university website, "The program offers a four-year, non-degree option for students with mild to moderate intellectual disabilities who want to actively engage in the full college experience, including participation in regular college classes, engaging in professional internships, and enjoying an active social life with friends." More information at *www.uc.edu*.

OUR EXPERIENCE: Public School to Community College

Overall, we have had some wonderful experiences during Dev's education. Sean and I believe in the philosophy of a free and appropriate education and we wanted all of our kids in the same system not just for convenience, but for equity. To that end, we have experienced several public systems. One was not an option because Devon would have been sent to a "special" school (not the neighborhood school). Inclusion is a top priority to our family. Another school failed even our typical children, the next went well until the economy plummeted, and the public school district we are in now is a work in progress . . .

What we have learned is that there are amazing teachers in terrible systems and there are deplorable teachers in amazing systems. At each step you have to re-evaluate, push, thank, explore, and team-build. It is not easy, but it is worth it.

Dev is about to move into a college setting as one of the first to be "dual-enrolled" in a contracted community college in our area. Keeping expectations high for our students and our systems is imperative; you never know if you do not try.

—SUE ADELMAN

Ruby's Rainbow

An organization that helps people with Down syndrome pursue their post-secondary education dreams is Ruby's Rainbow. Via their website, they remind families that "life and learning don't stop after high school. At Ruby's Rainbow, we want to help these amazing individuals with Down syndrome reach their highest potential." They do this by every year giving scholarships to individuals with Ds who are looking to continue their education post–high school. The list of "Rockin' Recipients" is growing; you may recognize a few. Check it out at *www.rubysrainbow.org*.

Other Post–High School Educational Opportunities

As with all young adults, college may or may not be the best option for your son or daughter's career goals and strengths. Be sure your child and her or his abilities and strengths are the center of the decision-making process. Also, be creative and open to making your own options. There are technical schools and community colleges, which can often be a part of the transition education process or even funded by vocational rehabilitation programs. There are also growing online options to consider in addition to specialized programs offered in your area for adults with developmental disabilities.

Some examples:

- In Omaha, Nebraska, there is a program run by The Ollie Webb Center, an affiliated chapter of The Arc, which offers continuing education in academics, life skills, and the arts.
- In North Texas there is an organization called My Possibilities, which serves the ongoing educational needs of adults with developmental disabilities from programs that teach how to "maintain and expand social skills, personal wellness, pre-vocational skills, and critical-thinking skills while becoming more involved in our community," on up to My Possibilities U, which includes training for specific industries, resume building, and career management classes.
- GiGi U is a program that is expanding locations throughout the country. It offers adults with Down syndrome classes to encourage health and wellness, career skills, and other areas of interest.

These are only a few examples of programs working today; there are many similar opportunities across the country.

It's commonly believed that typical adults today change careers an average of seven times. This may be in part because of economic changes, but not to be discounted is the fact that we, as humans, also change interests and goals over our lifetime. People with Down syndrome are no different in that regard. Throughout the lifespan of an adult with Down syndrome, it is important to keep offering learning experiences and personal growth opportunities.

Resources

- Think College: *www.thinkcollege.net*
- Your local college or university
- Ruby's Rainbow: *www.rubysrainbow.org*

Chapter Nine
Life for Adults with Down Syndrome

In this chapter we'll discuss the issues of adulthood with Down syndrome, including employment and housing options, the social lives and activities of adults, guardianship options, and future planning. We'll also look at medical conditions that are more common in adults with Down syndrome. Most of all, we'll hear the most important voices of this book, "My Stories"—adults with Down syndrome in their own words.

Dear New Parents,

You're on a quest for information, maybe even a crystal ball, trying to learn frantically about the future. A future that looks so different than the one imagined before . . . There is no crystal ball, you know. Your child, my child, they are each unique manifestations of the universe, and the next set of lists, suggestions, and decisions are so far away.

Yet, of course, adulthood arrives in a flash, ready or not. And, I *get* it. I know you have to read and devour and soak up the information for a while—I've been there. I hope this next chapter gives insight into some of the considerations, challenges, and opportunities that adults with Down syndrome live with today. Your child's future is not predicted in any of the following details. You know that, right? All right. Moving on.

Employment

"What are you going to be when you grow up?" Many of us, particularly Americans, place a heavy emphasis on vocation as part of our identity. Adults meeting each other for the first time often start the conversation with, "What do you do?" meaning, "What is your title and vocation?" Work and the value attributed to it are heavy indicators of social place and as such even parents of young children may already be worried about what a child with Down syndrome will grow up to *do*. As with so many programs involving people with varied abilities, this is an evolving prospect; so much has changed and improved over the last few years because of the work of advocates and self-advocates with even more strides regarding social and employment inclusion expected.

Employment Readiness

Just as for anyone else, opportunity for employment starts with proper education and training. Plus, your child's vocational goals may change several times as he grows from teenager to young adult (and beyond). Even so, all along the IEP process, consider and emphasize your child's interests and strengths with eventual employment options in mind.

Start with the essential building blocks of making social skills a priority. In the workplace the skills of listening, taking direction, and being respectful actually get an employee further down the road of security than almost anything else. Employees and prospective employees who are friendly and have a positive attitude consistently do better in a work environment. Consequently, do not minimalize the importance of including appropriate social skills in goal setting and as part of vocational training.

The next step is to build a resume. Just as in the case with the typical population, a variety of outside activities, volunteer work, and interests are all part of resume building. Encourage your teenager and young adult to explore and grow in a variety of areas in order to best prepare her for the work environment.

Where to Start

Most people with Down syndrome start working while in high school as part of their transition plan, and those who continue to a college program often also have job training as part of the curriculum (see Chapter 8). It is not unusual for high school students and young adults to begin gaining experience on a volunteer basis in their community. This is an important key to the resume building previously mentioned, as it not only develops skills but also connects your son or daughter to the community. Many high schools today require a certain number of "community hours" as part of graduation requirements as the lessons taught from volunteer work are just as, or more, critical to job training as academic skills.

Also during the transition process you may apply to your state's Department of Health and Human Services or Vocational Rehabilitation, and if needed, these programs will often provide the student with a job coach as she enters the workforce. Sometimes you may want to hire a job coach as a temporary measure. For example,

Marcus began a job in the bindery department of a print shop in his last year of school. A job coach accompanied him while he trained on the duties; after he was fully trained and the print shop felt comfortable with Marcus's progress, the job coach was no longer necessary. In other examples, a job coach may stay with an employee all the time while at a work site, and yet other times there may be a job coach who trains then merely "checks in" with both the employer and the employee to be sure all is well.

OUR EXPERIENCE: Beth's Job

Beth works at Little Caesars two evenings a week. She folds boxes, sometimes 300–400 in a three-hour span. According to her mother, Cindy, "She loves her job and the people she works with. The job coach stays with her until *Beth* is ready to work alone. The coach won't leave before then, even if she feels Beth is doing well enough; she waits until Beth feels confident enough to do the job alone. Then the job coach checks in occasionally. She also stays in regular contact with me and the store manager, making sure there are no issues that need to be addressed."

At this time there are also local, national, and international programs specifically designed to help adults with disabilities to find and acquire competitive employment. One example is Project SEARCH, an international program based out of Cincinnati, OH. Project SEARCH works to secure employment in the community for people with disabilities by creating programs with coaches, training, internships, and opportunity for inclusion and competitive wages in a variety of settings.

Apply

Another way self-advocates and families find employment is by asking and applying. Joey got a part-time job at age forty in his community barbershop when his nephew asked the owner to consider the match. All parties saw the benefits of having Joey working in the shop, and it led to a fifteen-plus-year ongoing job that brought a sense of worth and involvement to Joey, smiles to the clientele, and clean floors for the shop owner.

In the current employment market, companies are not required to give preference to people with disabilities; however, neither can companies discriminate against such people. The Americans with Disabilities Act means that employment discrimination is prohibited against "qualified individuals with disabilities." This means all persons, with or without Down syndrome, who can fulfill a job requirement can apply, be considered, and be employed for the jobs they are capable of working.

The American Dream

There are, as there always have been and will be, some people who would rather follow their own calling first and foremost. Down syndrome does not prevent the entrepreneurial spirit of adults in our community. There are adults with Ds who own and operate businesses from restaurants to apparel companies in addition to a growing number of artists, including jewelry, acting, and photography. Plus, sometimes the whole family gets involved like in J Ellen's House of Fabric, a quilting shop that employs people with developmental disabilities, where Sarah, a young woman with Down syndrome, is the "Sew-cial" Director.

Times Are Changing

There are still significant challenges regarding employment for adults with disabilities, according to the U.S. Department of Labor;

the unemployment and underemployment rate remains staggeringly high. Hopefully, the ABLE Act (discussed in Chapter 10) will ease restraints on employment options and empower adults to pursue bigger dreams.

Also, the landscape of fallback employment for many adults with developmental disabilities is currently in flux. As of April 2014, Disability Scoop reported that there are "an estimated 450,000 people with developmental disabilities nationwide currently spending their days in sheltered workshops and other segregated programs." These programs were designed to enable people with disabilities to have a day program that includes the satisfaction of employment, a token paycheck, and social interaction in a safe environment. Currently this model is undergoing drastic changes based on federal and state legislation. Although there will continue to be a need for those who cannot work competitively to have a safe day environment, it is unclear at this time what that work/training/care model will look like.

Right now both the government and private programs are encouraging both employers and communities to further explore the possibilities of working with people with Down syndrome, and sometimes that employer is the person with Down syndrome him/herself. The key along the way, throughout your child's education and beyond, is to focus on your offspring's strengths, be persistent in the community, and don't be afraid to get creative. As businessman Harry F. Banks said, "The secret of success is the consistency to pursue."

OUR EXPERIENCE: Josh's Employment

The first job Josh had was as a volunteer at our local humane society in the adoption center doing laundry, sweeping and mopping floors, as well as walking and playing with the dogs (and sometimes the cats). At that time we hired a job coach. His next job was assisting custodians at the school. Also volunteer work, but [he] gained a lot of experience! Then, the local zoo.

Next, Josh began working at a sheltered workshop, part-time. He attended school in the morning and worked in the afternoon. He loved it and also began collecting a paycheck, which he enjoyed tremendously! Working at the sheltered workshop provided Josh with so many positive experiences and opportunities to learn! This was his first paying job and again, he loved it. He was happy, fulfilled, and proud to have a job.

During the summer of 2014, Josh attended the summer school internship program offered by our school district. He had many responsibilities including meeting the young children who were being dropped off by their parents/guardians and helping them get to their classrooms safely. Josh also provided a courier service, delivering the afternoon attendance sheets to each of the bus monitors who worked at the program as paraprofessionals. During this program, Josh was next presented with the opportunity to work directly with a preschool classroom teacher, helping her in the day-to-day activities. Soon, he began to self-advocate. By the third week, Josh forcefully informed us, "I am going to work with the kids now!" With Josh, we presented this idea to the school system, and all agreed that it would be an excellent placement.

He is now a classroom helper at our local preschool with many responsibilities during his day that continue to evolve. This has been the first work placement of its kind in our school district! He is a volunteer, but the experience is priceless. He adores the children and is adored by them in return. He is a valuable member of the staff and is almost "all business" while he's there. His jobs get done with eagerness!

His coworkers tell us they feel a sense of joy when Josh is around and people often stop us when we visit to tell us something great about Josh and his experience in this work environment. Josh will be twenty years old in May 2015; we have no doubt that Josh will find gainful employment in a community-based company, because he is a valuable and hard-working employee who goes to work day in and day out, giving all that he has!

—KAREN GREGOIRE

Resources

- Institute for Community Inclusion: *www.communityinclusion.org*
- List of some of the people with Down syndrome who are business owners: *http://list.ly/list/OBK-businesses-by-adults-who-have-down-syndrome*
- Disability Benefits and Employment: *http://db101.org*
- Ticket to Work: *www.chooseworkttw.net*
- Project SEARCH: *www.projectsearch.us*

Housing

As adults with Down syndrome are living longer, fuller, more engaged lives, the options for living outside of the family home are also expanding.

According to the website of the American Society for Public Administration, "By the 2000s, K.C. Lakin and Roger Stancliffe (2007) identified four major trends in intellectual and developmental disabilities: decreasing use of institutions and increased use of housing; decreasing size among community settings; increasing numbers of people who live in homes they own or rent; and decreasing out-of-home placements of youth and children."

Where you live is a very personal decision. Having a Circle of Support and a person-centered plan, as briefly discussed in Chapter 8, allows and encourages self-advocates a voice in their living decisions. In addition to the considerations of cost, transportation, safety, and general availability of services, the wants and personality of the person with Down syndrome cannot be overlooked for his long-term health and happiness. The options for housing or living spaces are growing for adults with developmental disabilities and will continue to expand. Here are the most common current choices for people with Down syndrome.

With Family

It is still common for people with Down syndrome to live with their parents or a sibling as adults. The difference today from even twenty years ago is that this is a choice made together. Since there are so many other options at this time, this is most commonly taken by families who *want* to continue with the companionship, habits, and reliance upon each other. An article published on The Huffington Post, "Yes, My Adult Son with Down Syndrome Lives at Home," began, "The first thing you should know is this: My son Marcus is an adult with Down syndrome and he lives with us, not because he has to, but because we want to live together. Like millions, actually well over six million, [of] families with adult children who live 'at home' in the U.S. today, this is the best option for us right now." The most common comment reaction on the site and on the Facebook shares were sentiments like, "I wouldn't have it any other way," and "I can't imagine him/her anywhere else."

Parents and their adult children make this choice together, and thankfully it is one of many options to choose from. It is not unusual for siblings to also play a role in the home life of an adult with Down syndrome. (This is a decision the sibling should make with her family and never be an assumption or left to an emergency decision.) Also, there are families who have adjusted their once single-living homes to include an attached apartment, giving the adult with Ds a separate living space while still included in the parents' or sibling's family home. This option allows for varying levels of independence based on the adult child's needs and strengths.

MY STORY: CHARLEY PALMER

In a Skype interview, Charley Palmer shared his thoughts on his day-to-day life. His favorite day is Friday, because he stays home on the weekends. During the weekdays he attends the Sertoma Center, which offers community outings, a chance to work in the greenhouse, and activities, but truthfully, he'd rather just watch DVDs at home. Also, today he considered the greenhouse "hard work" (although we're told he doesn't feel like that every day). Charley is soon to be twenty-five and lives with his mom and dad. About the arrangement he says, "Yeah, still good." Charley's family has a strong social network of friends who will take Charley out to movies or just hang out with him. He loves his friends, and before the interview was over, he told me he loved me too, which is about the best way I've ever had an interview wrap up.

***

Host Family Living

An option similar to living with family, yet allows a person with Down syndrome to have his own space while still in a home environment, is to join a host family. Host families are most often engaged through a vendor that specializes in the housing and care of adults with developmental disabilities. The host family is trained and supported by a coordinator, and the company makes the suggested match between an individual and the host family. Although the setting may be similar to living with a person's own family, many adults find this option gives them further independence and learning opportunities, the self-esteem of having a home away from his parents, and depending on placement, more freedom and self-accountability.

Group Home

Group homes were the first step from the deinstitutionalization of people with disabilities. Since then, many organizations have striven to make residential group homes a comfortable and safe residential setting for adults with disabilities, with the goals of keeping the men and women involved in the community and encouraging a full, healthy life. Because the organizations care for several adults in one home, group homes offer daily living schedules that can be comforting to the adults who crave a structured day. Group homes also provide transportation to community events, outings, work and day centers, and sometimes medical visits. Group home staff is responsible for the meal preparation, medicine, and safety of the individual in the home, giving a sense of comfort to the family. Of course, not all group homes are "created equal." If you're contemplating this option, you should do extensive research before choosing a facility, including visiting, meeting administrators and staff, and checking references of the group home.

Community Cooperatives

There are also growing opportunities for people with disabilities to be a part of communities that partner with those with and without disabilities, each bringing their own talents and strengths to the group. One example is the Camphill Association of North America.

The organization's website, *www.camphill.org*, says, "Camphill in North America consists of ten independent communities that are home to over 800 people whose daily lives are full of vitality and accomplishment. These communities serve and impact thousands of other people in the surrounding areas. The ten communities live and work on over 2,500 acres of land, which is cared for utilizing organic and biodynamic methods."

The concept of people with and without disabilities working alongside each other is as natural as time itself. Marianne Robertson of the Fellowship for Intentional Community website described one such community: "Imagine a place where there is no discrimination and where everyone is treated with respect and has an opportunity to contribute. Innisfree is trying to create this kind of place in a village next to the Blue Ridge Mountains."

Thoughts from a Stranger

"I have an uncle with Down syndrome," the stranger told me. "Yeah, he lived with his mom till she died, then he moved to a group home."

"That must've been a shock," I replied. "How is he doing?"

"He loves the group home. He's taken over. It's 'his house' and he's become way more independent." Then he added, "I know she didn't mean to, but I think his mom's overprotection actually held him back."

Independent or Semi-Independent Space

Many adults with disabilities live in their own home space. These arrangements are often made with the help of family and range from duplex attachments to a home or apartment "across town." It is not unusual for adults to live with a friend or roommate, share expenses, and offset strengths. For example, one adult may be able to cook well and safely, whereas the other adult may help with laundry and other duties that make a household work. Whether alone, with a roommate, or even a spouse, sometimes another person may be contracted to check in on the adults and help in areas like medications, transportation, or daily living prompts.

Adults with Ds may qualify for rental assistance or low-income housing. The availability and requirements of these change from location to location. For an updated list of resources, check the U.S. Department of Housing and Urban Development (HUD) website, specifically under rental assistance, for more information on public housing, subsidized housing, and the Housing Choice Voucher Program (Section 8) options.

MY STORY: MICHAEL MCNALLY

Meet Michael McNally, a creative, hardworking young adult. His verbal language is difficult to understand. This does not mean he doesn't understand me, or anyone, or what is going on around him. We met before his book club meeting, where I learned, based on his language and gestures, they were just finishing up Pinocchio.

His mother joined us, so she could clarify his replies.

I explained to Michael that I was working on a book. "Can I ask you some questions?"

His spine straightened, his eyes lit up, and he leaned in. "Yes."

I asked permission to record the interview (important for details). He agreed and tested the sound by coughing, watching the recording line move. I started: "We're here talking to Michael McNally."

"That's right."

On what he likes to be called: "Friends call me Mikey."

On whom he lives with: "By myself."

Do you have a job? "Yes. North Sea Films studio. On Tuesday and Thursday."

Is that where you made your movies? "No."

Favorite day of the week: "Probably Monday."

With clarifications I learned that on Mondays, Mikey takes a sign language class and guitar lessons. He has directed five short films, one with another production company, Silver Screen in Omaha, where he also works part-time.

He plans to make a new zombie movie this summer. He was the assistant director to a Project Search film documentary; he did the storyboard and helped direct the shots. He's also working on a book called Help Me Be Good.

When he was younger he worked three years as a paperboy; he also cleans at the church.

Michael lives in an apartment by himself and is checked on by family and staff. There are other people in his apartment complex with learning disabilities, and they are encouraged to "hang out," have community classes on things like art, and cook dinners together.

His advice to new parents: "Hold your baby." And he added, "Send the mom flowers."

***

Changes

According to the U.S. Census Bureau, the average American moves 11.7 times in his or her lifetime. Keeping this in mind, circumstances will also change and adjustments will have to be made in the lives of adults with Down syndrome. Something you decide at the time your Ds offspring is entering young adulthood will probably not be the same ten or twenty years later. This is part of why enabling a child with Down syndrome to approach all her life decisions as a self-advocate will empower her to continue over a lifetime of decision-making points. The options for adults with Down syndrome will, no doubt, continue to expand, and you and your family should explore and embrace the variable opportunities as they arise.

The I-Word

Independence. Independence remains a loaded term in our society for parents of children with different abilities. It holds completely different meanings based on culture, family dynamics, and expectations. Also, the meaning evolves. For example, over the last World Down Syndrome Day weekend at a 321 eConference, Dr. Rekha Ramachandran, the co-founder and chairperson of the Down's Syndrome Federation of India (Tamil Nadu chapter) and president-elect of Down Syndrome International, reminded the attendees that, although she understands that "living independently" often infers in American culture living away from one's parents, for her having her daughter at home is natural, expected, and a blessing. This does not negate her daughter's contribution to their family dynamic, nor her independence in their community.

What does independent mean, anyway? For some families, independence means living outside of the parents' home, for some it means supported decision-making, and for some it means self-care.

In fact, as a person with Down syndrome ages, the I-word evolves from independence to individual. When people—you as parents, other family, friends, and ideally, the community—recognize a child, teen, and adult as his own individual, the I-word triumphs. What you will come to learn as your child reveals himself is the value of individuality. That I-word is the trump card over all the others.

Resources

This list is not an endorsement of these specific organizations but is provided to help you start your own research on available options and follow-up.

- The Mentor Network: *http://thementornetwork.com/program/host-home*
- Mosaic Info, Host Homes: *www.mosaicinfo.org/hosthomes*
- Developmental Disabilities Resource Center: *http://services.ddrcco.com/developmental-disabilities-services/residential-services*
- Camphill Association: *www.camphill.org*
- PACER Center, Housing Options: *www.pacer.org/housing/gettingstarted/housing-options.asp*
- The Arc, Housing Issues: *www.thearc.org/what-we-do/public-policy/policy-issues/housing*

Social Activities and Relationships in Adulthood

In the 1940s, psychologist Abraham Maslow created a pyramid of five basic and yet essential components to a person's optimal well-being. The base of this pyramid was composed of physiological needs, on which rested safety, followed by love/belonging, then esteem, and finally self-actualization. (This is called Maslow's Hierarchy of Needs.) These are the building blocks of a person's emotional wellness. The need for love and belonging, although abstract, impacts the concrete long-term effects in a person's health and happiness.

Challenges

Communication difficulties continue to make new relationships, in particular, challenging for adults with Ds. People with long-term friendships and family who understand a person's communication style are key to the social networks of adults who have difficulty with clear language. Some parents complain that their teenage or adult child with Ds prefers to surround herself in games, movies, and fantasy over the tangible interactions of human peers. This is not surprising if there are communication obstacles to sharing ideas about common interests.

As expressed in the Hierarchy of Needs, safety is an important issue; it is also a key challenge for adults with developmental disabilities. They may not have the skill set to maneuver safely on their own beyond certain physical or geographic boundaries, thus limiting their social interactions. Other adults with Ds, able to travel safely by means of public transportation or to facilitate their own rides to events, may not live in an area that has these options.

No matter the communication and social skills of a person with Ds, the need for friendship is tangible. As parents we need to help our children, throughout their lifetime, to have social interaction, to teach and encourage friendship, and to make this option available.

Dr. Karen Gaffney

Karen Gaffney is the first person with Down syndrome to swim in a relay team across the English Channel. She is the president of the Karen Gaffney Foundation, a public speaker, and a teacher, and in May of 2013, she received an honorary doctorate from the University of Portland. Through all of these accomplishments (of which I only listed the highlights; there are more), Dr. Gaffney confessed to the full auditorium of Best Buddies International, "The biggest challenge I faced when I was in school . . . It was not the long summers I spent in body casts recovering from five different surgeries. It was not extra time studying just to keep up with others in my class. It was not homework or tests. It was having friends. Good friends." (Watch the full video at *www.youtube.com/watch?v=_4kVTIBCV-o*; it's worth every minute.)

For this reason, Gaffney encourages students and adults to "reach out to someone who is different." One way she is working to help others to do this is through the Karen Gaffney Foundation "Friends First" Club, a project to facilitate students of different abilities working alongside each other on community projects. Thus they build companionship and make a difference in their neighborhoods and beyond.

Best Buddies International

The Best Buddies mission is "to establish a global volunteer movement that creates opportunities for one-to-one friendships, integrated employment, and leadership development for people with intellectual and developmental disabilities (I/DD)." The programs begin at middle school age, continue into adulthood, and include both social one-to-one friendships as well as supported employment opportunities. Best Buddies has chapters around the world and also has an e-Buddies program. Learn more about their programs at *www.bestbuddies.org*.

Programs such as these mentorships are great facilitators to inclusion of adults with Down syndrome in the wider community and the valuable lessons that friendship can teach people of all abilities.

Supported Programs

Some of the organizations within the I/DD and Ds communities that offer support and social programing for children continue on through adulthood. The Special Olympics works to help adults with disabilities to stay active and social in events around the world. These events are not all one-time, once-a-year opportunities. There are programs like bowling that last all year and are great segues into opportunities to participate in inclusive leagues as well. Across the United States there are a variety of options of sports to get involved with. Check out the program list to find what your state has to offer.

The Arc also has programs that cross the country with robust chapters that offer education, employment training, and placement, as well as social events. Many chapters sponsor dances, movies, and other projects that bring together folks with I/DD in safe and fun environments. (Find a chapter of The Arc and check out the calendar of events near you.) And, of course, check with your local DSA about social events for families of and adults with Down syndrome in your area.

The Next Chapter Book Club

"The mission of the Next Chapter Book Club is to provide meaningful opportunities for lifelong learning, social connections, and authentic community engagement for people with developmental disabilities through weekly book club meetings that include people with all reading levels." Book clubs are great opportunities for adults to meet new people and immediately have something in common to talk about. These book clubs are like any other book club, where people start by talking about the book and then sidetrack to talk about . . . whatever! The Next Chapter Book Club began in 2002, in Columbus, Ohio, and now has over 250 clubs in more than 100 cities located in twenty-nine states plus there are international clubs, too. Check out the website for information about your location or how to start a club in your area!

Facilitated Friendships

There are adults with Down syndrome, and adults with other I/DD, who spend most of the daytime in centers, with or without employment options available. Consequently, most of their time is spent in environments where the paid staff is their most consistent social interaction. Those adults who are unemployed or underemployed and whose families have arranged support for areas like transportation and respite, as well as people who live in group and even host homes, spend considerable time with a paid caregiver. These relationships have been called facilitated friendships and can include job coaches, staff at any day center or program, or any paid caregiver. A study by Rebecca Pockney with the University of Southampton discovered that most adults with a learning disability in that situation felt friendship toward the staff, even though the staff is what she terms "paid carers." Often, these people are the predominate source of social interaction for adults with learning disabilities. Although not common, in some cases, true friendships and "outside of work" social activities have followed. Since these arrangements are designed to be social and positive, these networks are just as important to the person with a disability as any other.

Inclusive Environments

Work is a top spot where adults of any ability make new friends. Sometimes workplaces promote further social activities that encourage interaction with coworkers. Be it annual events like the company picnic, employee-driven events like bowling leagues, or wellness activities like a walking club, joining in these events when possible offers great social opportunities.

Dating and Marriage

By now you've come to see and realize that people with Down syndrome have a full range of abilities and emotions. Naturally, when there is a "spark" between two people, there will hopefully be a date, then two, and then, who knows? Marriage?

The Talk

Talking to your children about puberty, hormone and physical changes, and sexuality is just as important with your child with Down syndrome as with any other child. Actually, maybe more so, because your child deserves to learn from a trusted source about both understanding physical changes and the desires associated, as well as appropriate boundaries for his or her long term well being. One helpful resource is *Teaching Children with Down Syndrome about Their Bodies, Boundaries and Sexuality: A Guide for Parents and Professionals* by Terri Couwenhoven; also, The Arc often hosts classes for teens and young adults about dating. Check your area.

In high school, there are often activities to encourage dating: school dances and other events. As your offspring ages into adulthood, school and work are still prime places to make new friends.

According to PewResearch.org, "Five percent of Americans who are in a marriage or committed relationship say they met their significant other online." Online dating is useful for people in what are called "thin dating markets," which includes people with disabilities. One new website that just recently opened online is a social networking platform specifically for people with disabilities: Special Bridge. It specifically helps adults with mental and physical disabilities to meet new people, up to and including romantic matching.

While this is an interesting and important option, most people still meet face to face, and romantic relationships are most often borne of long-term relationships.

OUR EXPERIENCE: Dating

Gina and her boyfriend have been dating for over a decade now. They have been friends since they were little. They live together in a nice apartment and they are so happy. Individuals with Down syndrome don't have to be defined by their disability. They can lead a normal productive life with proper support and guidance. My mom and I have always pushed her even when she feels like giving up (which does happen). Parents who are worried about their child's future have every right to be worried, but everything will work out fine.

—GINA'S BROTHER, JASON ROSS

Occasionally you will see a headline like "Couple shows people with Down syndrome can hold jobs, find love." Or "Sweethearts with Down syndrome to wed thirty years after meeting." These highlight the fact that people with Ds are active in their community, living longer, and are committed to loving relationships. The 2015 WDSD video "The Special Proposal" features the true-life story of one adult with Ds asking his girlfriend to move in with him. And the full-length documentary *Monica & David* shares not only the wedding but day-to-day living for this couple. Of course, as people with Ds and other learning disabilities continue to learn and work in the larger community, these stories will become less headline-worthy and more commonplace.

MY STORY: JENNY KOLEY

Jenny Koley is a receptionist at the Ollie Webb Center in Omaha, where she has worked for five years. She is a thirty-five-year-old self-advocate. I asked about her life outside of work and what's next.

On living with her parents: "I love it, yeah." (Later in the conversation, I learned Jenny has a basement apartment in the house.)

On outside of work activities: "I like to act. I also like bowling. I'm on a league. Also, I like bocce ball and Camp Luther."

On making friends: "I'm part of a book club; I make friends there. Also I make friends at work."

On serving a two-year term on the board of her local DSA: "I was able to follow my dream: to speak up for myself, and to speak up for others."

On what's next: "Other than working here... I kind of want to start my own acting business. I'm getting experience taking acting classes. I want to work more with training [other actors]."

On what she wants the world to know: "My motto is live your life. Enjoy your friends. Enjoy work."

On advice to parents: "Love your kids. And, let your children make their own decisions."

At the end of the interview she added: "I want to say one more thing: My parents are my inspiration. Also, my acting teacher, Jim [Hoggat]. They are very supportive of my dreams."

***

Resources

- Best Buddies: *www.bestbuddies.org*
- "Friends First" Club: *www.karengaffneyfoundation.com*
- Special Olympics: *www.specialolympics.org/Regions/north-america/_Region-Front/North-America.aspx#ProgramList*

- Next Chapter Book Club: *http://nextchapterbookclub.org*
- The Arc Program for Adults: *www.thearc.org/find-a-chapter*
- Special Bridge: *www.specialbridge.com*

www.connectwc.org/dating-relationships-sexuality.html

- Disability Scoop, Dating 101: *www.disabilityscoop.com/2008/12/15/dating101/5186*

Guardianship and Future Planning

What is more daunting than the future? Nothing, because, of course, you have no real control over it. Documentation is the best thing parents can do to prepare for their child's future. Note: The options listed here are for informational purposes only and do not constitute legal advice. We're offering these opinions to show the diversity of options and information available to you and your offspring.

Beginning Future Planning

The Letter of Intent (LOI) introduced in Chapter 4 does not replace the legally binding documentation of a will, but it is the first step to letting your family and yes, the state, know what the plan is for your child with disabilities. It also gives important information regarding their health needs and daily living. It's less daunting than the work, thought, and expense required for a will. That said, if the phrase "ward of the state" concerns you in any way, it's time to invest in a will. If you don't have a will, then upon your death the state will have no direction regarding your wishes about the guardianship of your children and the distribution and management of your estate. Consider contacting an attorney who is experienced with special needs planning; check with the Special Need Alliance for an attorney in your area and talk to other parents in your area and get referrals.

Note to Parents

Mortality is hard. No one wants to face it. Gathering people together to make a long-term plan and put it in place may sound stressful; however, it actually reduces parental, and your family's, anxiety for the future.

The Arc Center for Future Planning

The Arc Center for Future Planning is a user-friendly, online, step-by-step tool to help families get started and follow through with long-term plans. It's important to remember, making a plan for the future, in and of itself does not cost any money. Do not neglect the importance of documentation, talking to your family, and making a long term plan because you feel that you are not financially able to take these steps. Use the free resources, like the checklists and educational webinars that are offered on The Arc's Future Planning website. Most of the process is about communication within your family and enabling your son or daughter to be a part of the process. Give yourself peace of mind by starting early.

Age of Majority

As a person with Down syndrome reaches the age of majority, which is eighteen in most U.S. states, your self-advocate and your family will need to decide on the best way to legally handle decisions regarding medical issues, handling financial responsibilities, and capacity for understanding and signing contract agreements and other legal documents. Many parents have defaulted to legal guardianship as the only option. In recent years this has shifted, however, to allow for other legal safety nets that are less intrusive on rights of the person with disabilities and are based on his or her capacity to make decisions. At this time, the primary legal options for most states are medical power of attorney, power of attorney, and traditional guardianship. The laws, requirements, and restrictions on each of these vary from state to state.

Considerations Regarding Guardianship

The first thing to consider is, of course, the level of understanding and responsibility of the Ds adult to make informed decisions, balanced against the wants of the person to be under the care of another person or to be emancipated. The second thing to consider is what rights the person will be giving up as a ward. According to the Guardianship.org document "Rights of an Individual under Guardianship": "The court should specifically state which rights it is taking from the ward. The ward keeps all rights that the court has not specifically given to the guardian." Additionally, every state has different laws that apply to those who are under guardianship; for example, in New Jersey, people with a legal guardian are not allowed to marry.

Another consideration that varies from state to state is the right to vote once a person is under guardianship. Some states allow for limited guardianship, or special requests or inquiries regarding voting, and some are "blanket rulings."

About Guardianship

Your biggest concern if you're considering guardianship should be your child's safety and medical information and needs. In the booklet entitled *Do I Need a Guardian for My Family Member Who Has Down Syndrome?* compiled for the Down Syndrome Guild of Greater Kansas City by Craig C. Reaves, CELA, of Reaves Law Firm, P.C., the suggested rule is: "If your family member who has Down syndrome has sufficient mental capacity to live on his or her own, make appropriate decisions and manage his or her money, then a durable power of attorney should be signed by your family member to forestall the necessity of appointing a guardian if your family member loses this mental capacity. This is no different than for every adult, including you.

If, on the other hand, your family member does not have sufficient mental capacity, then guardianship should be pursued in order to make sure your family member is adequately protected." Ultimately, a person has to be "of sound mind" (that is, understand the issues and consent) in order to grant a legally binding power of attorney.

Different states offer different levels of guardianship options, as well. Some states have what's called limited guardianship, which only applies to certain areas. Also, some states have a "guardian advocate." This may allow for more individual rights—for example, in Florida, if a person has a guardian advocate, she or he is allowed to vote. Kansas, as another example, has a Plan of Guardianship option, which spells out what rights the ward is allowed to retain and is approved by the courts. In many states, all legal rights are removed unless the guardianship order specifically reserves the authority for the ward. Perhaps it is because of these wide variations in state laws, moving a person under guardianship from state to state can require additional paperwork and a fresh review of the situation, including a review in court. The Uniform Law Commission is working with legislators to make the process of state-to-state moves simpler.

Choosing the Responsible Parties

Once you've decided on the best legal model for the adult with Down syndrome, you must choose the person or persons to be the legal guardian, have power of attorney, or be the financial conservator and/or social support. Make this decision early, involving your Circle of Support. This decision can, and likely will, change over the years. Sometimes duties are split between a guardian and a conservator, and sometimes there are co-guardians. Some states require, particularly if there are sufficient assets, a guardian and a conservator (for financial responsibility). When building a team for your child's circle of support, consider the variety of roles that need to be filled for your child's future care.

This decision is not one to be made in an emergency or under pressure. All parents, regardless of the number of children, should discuss support options for their child early and often.

OUR EXPERIENCE: Taking Care of Sister

Evonne is my older sister, five years older. The earliest memory I have of Evonne is her laughing and always playing with us. After my parents divorced, I felt I had to be in charge of making sure my sisters were taken care of.

As an adult, Evonne lived at home for a few years then eventually moved to a group home in Amarillo. In 2011, she fell in front of her group home and broke her arm and her foot. She had surgery and went through rehab at a nursing home. She was allowed to go back home (to the group home) after her healing had her almost back to normal. She regularly sees her doctors (general practitioner, oncologist, psych, etc.) and the group home does a wonderful job of making sure she gets where she needs to go and making sure she has everything she needs.

Since our parents died, I am her guardian advocate, which is not the same as guardian. Since she has a legal advocate, she is her own guardian and makes her own legal decisions. This is my understanding from talking to social workers, doctors, and group home staff. I was kind of defaulted into this position. I went in blind.

I average a trip to her every other month, sometimes once a month. I speak to her on the phone probably three or four times a week. The staff at her group home contacts me if something is needed.

—ANGIE BOGGS

Helping Adult Siblings Get Started

The National Down Syndrome Congress (NDSC) has recently released an online Adult Siblings Packet to help gather information, start discussions, and consolidate important planning and day-to-day details. Although the packet title is specific to siblings, the information to gather and think about is helpful for any caregiver situation. Check it out here: *www.ndsccenter.org/adult-siblings*.

A Siblings Study done by the Easter Seals showed that siblings often feel unprepared for the role of caregiver, even if they expect to take on that responsibility. Also, while they are concerned particularly about the financial implications, they are commonly unaware of the various resources available to them and their loved one. As parents, please include as part of your future planning the details, resources, and information you have learned over the years and be sure it is documented and ready to be shared with the next person to step into the caregiver role for your child with Down syndrome.

Supported Decision-Making

In 2013 a woman with Down syndrome named Jenny Hatch won a legal case to change guardianship from her parents. Her case made national headlines and is the foundation for the Jenny Hatch Justice Project. Groups that advocate for those with disabilities, and others, praised the decision. Susan Mizner of the American Civil Liberties Union said this case should be a reminder that "supported decision-making and providing powers of attorney are the options we should look to first—rather than reflexively choosing guardianship and stripping a person of every civil liberty."

From Article 12 of the United Nations Convention on the Rights of Persons with Disabilities

"With supported decision-making, the presumption is always in favour of the person with a disability who will be affected by the decision. The individual is the decision-maker; the support person(s) explain(s) the issues, when necessary, and interpret(s) the signs and preferences of the individual. Even when an individual with a disability requires total support, the support person(s) should enable the individual to exercise his/her legal capacity to the greatest extent possible, according to the wishes of the individual."

The legal landscape for people with Down syndrome and independence continues to evolve. This is why you should investigate all options and involve the self-advocate in your life before making any legal decisions. Document, detail, and discuss the decisions in order to help and protect everyone involved.

MY STORY: AMANDA BAILEY

Amanda is forty-four years old and currently lives with her brother and his wife. Amanda had to self-advocate to include her wishes in a guardianship court battle that ended in what she called "Freedom Day." She and her sister, Nancy Bailey, wrote about this experience in the recent release, The North Side of Down.

In summary, Amanda's father and guardian thought he had made his wishes for her future clear and believed that she would be safely cared for by her older brother, Ted. Unfortunately, the legalities of this transition were not handled in detail before his death, thus embroiling the family in a legal battle that was nothing less than traumatic, compounded by the fact it immediately followed the death of their father.

About the book, Amanda stated, "We tell it like it is!"

"Yes we do! And hopefully it will help someone else," Nancy added.

"I hope so, too," Amanda agreed.

Nancy impressed that, "People with disabilities need to have a voice." And, "It is important for people (caregivers) to get their affairs in order, to make their wishes known in a legal, undisputable way . . . and that real love can withstand anything."

Amanda also shared:

On writing: "I journal every day. I guess I write about the family [and] what I do during the day. I write at night and in the morning. I [also] like to write letters."

On another book: "I am *working on another book."*

On her new home: "I love it here."

On friends: "It's kind of hard to make new friends. But I have made great, wonderful friends who are good to me. We swim together, have bible study, and go to church on Sunday."

On advice to new parents: "Don't do drugs, smoking, or drinking. And put them [your child] in Special Olympics."

***

Resources

- Letter of Intent: *www.scribd.com/doc/251683759/First-Steps*
- National Caregivers Library: *www.caregiverslibrary.org*
- The Arc Center for Future Planning: *https://futureplanning.thearc.org*
- NDSC Siblings Packet: *www.ndsccenter.org/adult-siblings*

- Attorneys specializing in special needs: Special Needs Alliance: *www.specialneedsalliance.org*
- National Guardianship Association: *www.guardianship.org*
- Got Transition, Guardianship Alternatives: *www.gottransition.org/resources/index.cfm#guardianshipanddecisionmaking*
- The Jenny Hatch Justice Project: *http://jennyhatchjusticeproject.org*
- National Resource Center for Supported Decision-Making: *http://supporteddecisionmaking.org*

Medical Considerations in Adulthood

As your child with Down syndrome ages, her medical needs and providers will change. Many children with Ds see a pediatrician for their health needs, and as is the custom, will have to move on to a general practitioner, or a Ds specialist, as she ages into adulthood. The first issue important to the care of adults with Down syndrome is "continuity of care."

Continuity of Care

Continuity of care means establishing a team of consistent caregivers that includes your child's medical professionals and other service providers, all with access to medical history and current care information, and the approach of clear communication between specialists, general medical professionals, and caregivers. This methodology both prevents problems through cooperative monitoring of the patient's well-being and is actually found most cost effective because of the preventative and cooperative nature of the communication. Clinics that specialize in serving children and adults with Down syndrome generally adhere to this thinking as best practice, however you may not live near or in an area with a Ds clinic. In this case, it is up to you to facilitate a medical team that will share records and communicate any concerns about your child's health and wellness. Discuss how to facilitate continuity of care with your general practitioner while your child is still a teenager and prepare your child's medical transition plan as they age. Transition planning should begin in the mid-teenage years for medical care as it does for education planning.

Because of the varied challenges the population of people with Ds face, including communication difficulties, continuity of care is a crucial component to the mental and physical well-being/overall health of adults with Ds. That said, it's not always easy to attain, and like every other chapter of your child's life, requires certain diligence and planning.

It's Complicated

Perhaps more than any other area, the medical needs of the people in the Down syndrome community vary in extremes, and each person is particularly unique in the way that trisomy 21 manifests itself from person to person.

Consequently, when obtaining a physician to care for an adult with Ds, it is important they are equipped with the general guidelines for common challenges of the medical needs of people with Ds, but also acknowledge specific symptoms of the individual and respect the self-advocate's opinions, needs, and voice. Just as there may be doctors and specialists who discount treatable conditions in children with Ds, it is critical to remain diligent with the needs and treatment of the adults in the Ds community as well.

OUR EXPERIENCE: Find the Right Care

Michael is fifty-three, so yes, many times over many years, there have been treatments ignored or not even started due to the existing diagnosis of Ds. I move on immediately. This might be more difficult for those in small rural areas with limited medical, but for us, the only option is to move on.

So many different types of parents. Some want to make a big issue of this. Not worth it to me. We move on to another professional, well-managed health-care provider. Know what is best for your child and you, and stay with that doctor (specialist). When not right, move on.

If you recognize a huge issue with missed—or not willing to [provide]—care for a child/adult with Ds—report it. Report to medical boards, hospital[s], etc., and in any case, move on.

—MARY WASSERMAN

Available on the NDSS website is a list of health-care guidelines for adults with Ds. These guidelines are based on 1999 guidelines and are clearly in need of an update, but they're an appropriate starting point to share with your physicians.

Adults with Down Syndrome Task Force

The Global Down Syndrome Foundation (GDSF) has created an adult task force committee that has among its goals to update the medical care guidelines for adults with Down syndrome.

Also, on the GDSF website is a map of medical centers across the country that have one or more doctors specializing in the care of persons with Down syndrome.

OUR EXPERIENCE: Aging

Aging is a difficult topic. We don't like to think about ourselves being negatively affected by Father Time, let alone our children. In the Down syndrome community, it's the least talked about stage of life. We all know the main reason: our children are living longer now than ever before. There just isn't as much information out there. Pressure to stay positive about Down syndrome limits the spaces where we can have honest, open discussions about caring for our adult and aging children.

But think about that—our children are *living longer*. Yes, there may be bumps in the road but it's up to us to learn how to best support them, however uncomfortable it may be for us to think about.

—STEPHANIE HOLLAND, FOUNDER OF *THE ROAD WE'VE SHARED*

Following is a brief overview of some of the most common manageable conditions that adults with Down syndrome may face. The information provided is intended to be informative and educational and is not a replacement for professional medical evaluation, advice, diagnosis, or treatment by a health-care professional.

Common Physical Challenges

- **Atlantoaxial Instabilities (AAI):** It is suggested that children with Down syndrome receive x-rays to diagnosis atlantoaxial (spinal) instabilities that result from increased flexibility between the first and second bones of the neck. Some people have developed AAI after the initial screening in childhood, so you should re-screen once each decade. If your child or adult is going to have surgery, he should also be screened before any surgery that will involve the use of a breathing tube since there have been reports, although rare, of neck injury during placement of the breathing tube.

- **Osteoporosis and osteoarthritis:** Osteoporosis and osteoarthritis are each more common in adults with Down syndrome than in the general population. Calcium supplementation of 1,000 mg for men and nonmenopausal women and 1,500 mg for postmenopausal women (along with vitamin D) may help to reduce/prevent symptoms of reduction of bone density. Also, as with the typical population, the best way of preventing these conditions is to lead an active lifestyle. If an adult with Down syndrome has previously been active and begins to resist activity, be sure to address the possibility that pain may be an issue, and discuss with your doctor.
- **Cardiac:** Half of adults with Down syndrome have cardiovascular concerns. The most common are acquired mitral valve prolapse (MVP) and valvular regurgitation. An echocardiogram can easily diagnose each issue, so you'll want to consult a cardiologist about regular monitoring.
- **Eyes:** Cataracts occur in up to 13 percent of persons with Down syndrome. Keratoconus occurs in up to 15 percent, and 25 to 43 percent of these persons have refractive error. You need to schedule regular vision examinations in order to identify age-related changes and other pathological eye conditions.
- **Ears:** Adults with Down syndrome tend to experience hearing loss more often and earlier than the typical population. The NDSS suggests periodic screening with an audiologist to formally assess hearing issues and address concerns that can be treated, such as wax impactions, and the need for or maintenance of assistive devices like hearing aids.
- **Skin Issues:** Most skin conditions common in adults with Down syndrome can be managed under the care of a dermatologist or your regular physician via antibiotic creams, or sometimes an oral prescription is necessary to combat infections. People with Ds are also more likely than the general

population to have alopecia, an immune deficiency disorder that results in hair loss as one of its symptoms. A few treatment options are available to adults that are not available to children. However, these treatments have notable side effects or pain to consider.

- **Sleep Apnea:** Basically, sleep apnea is when a person stops breathing while asleep. There are three types of sleep apnea: obstructive, central, and mixed. Of the three, obstructive sleep apnea, often called OSA for short, is the most common. According to the NDSS, over half of all people with Down syndrome experience obstructive sleep apnea. Sleep is important to the body's ability to recover; it mends itself, and regulates blood pressure during sleep. Those are important to overall health and well-being, but not breathing causes serious long- and short-term negative effects on the body and the brain. Physicians now suggest all children with Down syndrome should be screened for sleep apnea by age four and regular check backs are also important. A complete sleep study provides the definitive information when there is a concern based on symptoms. Also, over time, the treatments often need to be adjusted.
- **Thyroid:** Between 10 percent and 40 percent of adults with Down syndrome are diagnosed with hypothyroidism, which means the thyroid gland is underactive and does not make enough thyroid hormone. Hyperthyroidism, the other extreme, where the thyroid makes too much thyroid hormone, also has a higher incidence in the Ds community. Undiagnosed hypothyroidism can contribute to dementia or be misdiagnosed as dementia. Adults with Ds should be tested annually to track and adjust the effects of thyroid issues. With prescription medication and also adjusted diet and exercise, these issues are easily managed.

Common Mental Challenges

- **Anxiety/OCD/Depression:** Adults with Down syndrome are certainly not immune to anxiety, difficulty processing emotional trauma, and related issues. It is important for parents and families to understand that the discomfort, even mental pain, caused from generalized anxiety, OCD, and depression are real and that millions of Americans struggle with these challenges.

Important to note: Sometimes symptoms corresponding to mental health come about because of a physical manifestation; for example, thyroid issues or hearing loss may lead to less ability to interact, which can look like brain fog, stubbornness, or depression. Once physical medical conditions are ruled out, your doctor can treat a person with Down syndrome's mental wellness or refer you to further professionals like a therapist, psychologist, or psychiatrist.

Alzheimer's Disease

This is a significant concern that affects people with Down syndrome more commonly, and earlier, than the general public so it's worth discussing this separately from other conditions.

Common early symptoms of Alzheimer's disease include short-term memory loss, frequent confusion, a change in interest in activities, or becoming withdrawn or frequently frustrated with conversation. In terms of behavior, a person may start wandering or losing his ability to find his way or he may begin forgetting how to handle household tasks that were previously mastered, like using a microwave or making coffee. Sometimes adults with Down syndrome begin to have seizures as a early indicator of the disease.

Alzheimer's disease is a diagnosis that carries emotional weight. So here are brief notes of what we know, what we don't know, and what we hope.

What we know: For those of us in the typical population Alzheimer's disease occurs in as much as 75 percent in people after the age of sixty-five. For people with Down syndrome, there are three additional factors:

- People with Down syndrome experience accelerated aging, meaning they tend to show the physical symptoms of aging in adulthood an average of fifteen years before the typical population.
- Recently the connection between the twenty-first chromosome and the APP gene (amyloid beta (A4) precursor protein) has been discovered. The APP gene, put simply, plays a strong role in the development of Alzheimer's disease effect on the brain.
- A person with Ds is more likely to develop Alzheimer's before the age of sixty-five.
- The brain of a person with Ds is predisposed to significant levels of the protein, plaques, and tangles that occur in people with Alzheimer's. In fact, by the age of forty nearly everyone with Down syndrome will develop these physical manifestations.

"Despite this, just over half (of people with Ds) have clinical evidence of dementia, and many living beyond 70 will never develop clinical AD." From "Screening for Alzheimer's Disease in Downs Syndrome" by Rónán O'Caoimh, Yvonne Clune, and D. William Molloy.

What we don't know: Why doesn't everyone with Down syndrome get Alzheimer's when the physiological manifestation of plaques and tangles are there? Why do some people with Ds show signs as early as age thirty-five and half of those with Ds never show signs of Alzheimer's at all?

What we hope: That scientists are right now on track to cure Alzheimer's disease, for people with Down syndrome as well as the typical population.

Health Challenges You Didn't See on This List

Yes, the list of challenges that adults with Ds are predisposed to is unnerving. Here's some good news: There are a few conditions that a person with Ds is *very unlikely* to experience: high blood pressure, heart attacks, or hardening of the arteries. Also, with the exception of a rare pediatric leukemia, even elderly adults with Down syndrome rarely develop solid tumors.

Lifestyle and Wellness

We cannot stress enough the importance of self-advocacy on health and wellness issues. Adults with Down syndrome can and do make their own healthy habits and changes when given the education and opportunity to do so. Making healthy choices as a family is important. That said, parents have been known to find that their child (adult or younger) with Ds actually makes healthier choices than the parents, *given the option*. Encourage the other "teachers" in her life, like doctors, dentists, and workout instructors, to explain the health and lifestyle benefits to making healthy choices, and prepare to allow the self-advocate in your life to change and stick to good habits.

NOTE FROM THE AUTHOR

This really should be titled a confession from the author. Habit-changing is hard. *Hard*. Among my parental regrets, and we all have a few, is how many bad eating and inactivity habits I instilled into my son while he was a child. Work, school, and life take time, but fast food, processed foods, and pop (soda, or whatever carbonated beverages are called in your part of the country) are never, never, *never* good for the endocrine system, the skin, the brain, or any component of my son's well-being—or me. In learning the true risks to our health, realizing the capacity for the long-term effects on our quality of life, we swallowed hard and now recognize the toxins when we see them. We slowly began to make changes, and we're not perfect.

My son has been a partner in these changes and helps to keep us in line. We used to be heavy pop drinkers, but one day he got in the car and said, "I'm not drinking pop anymore."

Then he marched into his workout and told his friends the same.

This was a few years ago and he drinks a soda very rarely, still. Based on his own declaration.

I can see the benefits to his well-being with each new change. I wish I began teaching him about healthy foods and habits when he was younger, but regret doesn't burn any calories. I know that with every positive change we make today there will be more potential for a better tomorrow, so we move forward to do better one step at a time.

—Mardra

As with every other human being on the planet, staying active, eating well, not eating junk, being socially active, and getting good sleep are critical to improving outcomes for healthy living for people with Ds. Do not negate the importance of these actions at every life stage.

Some reminders and tips:

- **Immunity-boosting foods:** People with Down syndrome need to boost their immune system. Antioxidant foods such as strawberries, raspberries, and blueberries are all yummy and healthy choices. The Mayo Clinic suggests *shopping the perimeter* when you go to the store. Stick to the freshest food available when filling the grocery cart by avoiding the center aisles that are filled with processed, boxed, salted, and sugary foods.
- **Fish is brain food:** According to ALZinfo.org, "A diet rich in fish, particularly oily fish like tuna, salmon, mackerel, sardines, and anchovies, may lower the risk of Alzheimer's disease and other forms of dementia." The article goes on to say that using supplements of fish oil containing DHA and other omega-3s is also beneficial.
- **Stay social:** Dr. William Mobley, professor and neuroscientist, in addition to Dr. Dennis McGuire, a specialist in the care of adults with Down syndrome, have both emphasized in public speeches the importance of staying socially active to the well-being of the brain and the body.
- **Sleep:** Do not underestimate the importance of good sleep for the body and the brain.
- **Water:** Proper hydration is critical to digestion, expelling toxins, skin health, oxygenating the brain, and weight loss. It's probably the easiest and cheapest way to improve your health. Drink plenty of water.
- **Physical activity:** No matter the challenges, nothing can replace the long- and short-term benefits of physical movement. More than weight loss, which is important to the overall health of many adults with Down syndrome, there are also psychological benefits of endorphins and brain benefits of increased oxygen.

OUR EXPERIENCE: Get Creative

Today, when we took the old champ to our lodge for his spa shower, [we] saw a posting for a new class we know he'll enjoy. Chair dancing! He's been wheelchair dancing for a long while. Now he can add chair dancing class with his neighbors. This is a great addition to his chair yoga class. All fitness here is directed by a professional trainer, so some workout is guaranteed. We're busy staying active in our 55+ community.

—MARY WASSERMAN

Everyday Active

Here are some ideas for everyone in the family to help stay active. Note: When your adult son or daughter doesn't live with you, you can still encourage and join in on many of these activities. If there are people assisting with your child's life skills, make sure everyone is on board that preventative healthcare is just as much of a priority as emergency health care. Remember, everything counts!

- Encourage getting up during all commercials: Take a "race in place," do jumping jacks, walk the stairs, or dance together.
- Jumping on a rebounder (a small trampoline) even five minutes a day oxidizes blood and can even improve mood. Have your son jump to 3 or 4 of his favorite songs.
- Take a class once a week: Anything—dance, yoga, cardio, strength, whatever. This can be with a certified gym/health club or at the local college, The Arc, or often the YMCA. Not only good for the family but also a great way to stay active in your community.

- Park at the end of the lot instead of at the front—make it a rule to return the cart to the inside of the store.
- Choose a restaurant/coffee shop you can walk or ride your bike to together.
- Zoo member? Walk there. It is safe and fun. Some zoos even have walking clubs that will welcome your adult son as part of the club.
- Facilitate walking dates with friends/family. Get everyone on board!

Caring for the Caregiver

Just as in Chapter 1 when we emphasized the need to care for yourself, the same is true throughout the lifespan of your children. Healthy habits you adopt as a family lead to a better, longer, more fulfilled quality of life. You need to make and take time for yourselves, and be a good example for your children (at any age).

OUR EXPERIENCE: Joshua's Advice to a New Parent

I wanted to tell Holly's friend, who just had a baby with Down syndrome, "Oh, how wonderful for them!" Sure, I know some of the struggles that are ahead. These young parents are not in the same place I am now . . . because, with age comes a lot of perspective. Oh, people sometimes call it "wisdom," but I call it "time." And "learning from my mistakes." And, "learning to see the big picture." These young ones? Well, I'm sure they are feeling many emotions.

Things are more different now than even just twenty-nine years ago, when I had Joshua. There seems to be more knowledge . . . more acceptance of . . . more services for . . . kids with Ds.

I warmed up some "reruns" for Joshua's lunch. That's what he calls "leftovers." I decided to see what he would have to say about the situation with Holly's friend, and I tried to prepare myself for anything he might say. I wanted him to say his honest opinions.

I said, "Hey, Joshua . . . a friend of Holly's just had a brand-new baby boy . . . and he has Down syndrome, like you!"

He said, "Oh, wow!"

"What do you think about that?"

"That's a pretty good kid if he came out like that," he said.

I asked him if he had any advice for the new parents and he asked, "What advice did you get when you had me?"

I told him how my friend came over to visit after we brought him home from the hospital . . . about how she sat on our couch and held him while we talked. She told me, "Just love him."

I thought, "Well, that's easy! Look how cute he is!"

(Joshua just grinned and grinned when I said that part.)

Joshua said, "I'll go with that, too. Love him. And train him up to be a man of God."

Then he started quoting scripture after scripture at me, and I could not even keep up. He ended his sermon talk with these words: "I turned out okay, and he will, too."

—JOSHUA'S MOM, MARTY GARLAND ORIGINALLY PUBLISHED ON MARTY'S MOOSE TRACKS: *HTTP://MARTYSMOOSETRACKS.BLOGSPOT.COM*

Resources

- Disability.Gov Caregiver's Guide: *www.disability.gov/resource/disability-govs-guide-family-caregivers*

- American Family Physician, Health Care for Adults with Down Syndrome: *www.aafp.org/afp/2001/0915/p1031.html*
- NDSS Adult Health Care Guidelines: *www.ndss.org/Resources/Health-Care/Health-Care-Guidelines/Adult-Health-Care-Guidelines*
- GDSF map of medical providers: *www.globaldownsyndrome.org/research-medical-care/medical-care-providers*
- AlzInfo.org: *www.alzinfo.org*

Part Three
YOU ARE NOT ALONE

Chapter Ten
Down Syndrome Support and Research

We have introduced you to several of the Down syndrome organizations that are available to support and advocate for and with families of children and adults with Down syndrome. This chapter details the purpose of the local and national groups, and how to find and reach them.

Dear New Parents,

As mentioned in Chapter 1, participation is voluntary. One group, all groups, or no groups: It's all about you and your family. The first point of contact between you and "the community," with comfort, advice, and contacts to help you navigate the systems and find answers often begins with the local organization. As you begin this new adventure, the local, national, and international groups all aim to support you and your family. How this looks is unique to each group's mission and to your needs. We hope you will find comfort in knowing the work so many are doing to improve the lives of our children and provide new connections and resources.

Local Organizations

Local groups are the frontline of support for families and self-advocates. The local Down Syndrome Association (DSA) often hosts support events for moms, dads, and extended family. Also, they advocate in local politics on issues that affect people with Down syndrome and their families, as well as raise awareness and acceptance in the community. Local groups are often affiliates of a national organization, meaning they both garner and give support to a nationally based Down syndrome organization. These partnerships are mutually beneficial as the local group can benefit from the years of experience and recognition a national group brings.

Support has its place at every stage of a person's life.

OUR EXPERIENCE: Local Groups

My son is seven weeks old, [and] this group [the Rio Grande Valley Down Syndrome Association] has been helpful as I have been able to ask questions about what to expect in regard to development and milestones. It's also very nice to have a group of people who understand what you are going through and who offer their support all day every day. They have been great!!

—CHRISTINA BOTELLO

Links to Find a Local Group

If you need help finding a local Down syndrome group, check the National Down Syndrome Society for a local affiliate: *www.ndss.org/Resources/Local-Support*. The Global Down Syndrome Foundation has a listing at *www.globaldownsyndrome.org/about-down-syndrome/resources/local-organizations*.

OUR EXPERIENCE: Cincinnati Down Syndrome Association

Greater Cincinnati DSA (dsagc.com) has great parent, family, and teacher information to share, PT and OT group sessions for nothing or almost nothing (birth to five), music therapy for minimal (ten weeks for $20), adult classes in dance and independent living, meetings on medical issues, meetings for parent panels of discussion, meetings to explain some of the therapies, meetings to talk about legislation and financial information, play groups by region and or year, DADS (Dads Appreciating Down Syndrome) group, Mom's night out by region, family picnic, holiday party and other social events, lending library with lots of books and now iPads, great people in the office, plus Cincinnati has a children's hospital with a Ds clinic.

We also have one of the largest (if not largest) Buddy Walks in the nation (11,000 people minimum) with food, vendors, games, music, bounce houses, arts and crafts projects, performance[s] by several of the group classes, and some great support from the teams and clubs that have included our kids. All of this for free (except vendors do sell a few things), with ages ranging from pre-birth to sixty-plus years old."

—MARY PATRICK

Sometimes it is difficult for people in remote areas to have this same sort of inclusion and support; fortunately through the Internet there are a growing number of connections and shared education. Online communities are holding an increasingly important role in supporting parents and will be discussed further in Chapter 11.

Down Syndrome Affiliates in Action

Another group helps both the local groups and national organizations. Called the Down Syndrome Affiliates in Action, it has a mission, as it says, to "support and advance the growth and service capabilities of the local and regional Down syndrome organizations we serve, to be the conduit of value-driven training, programs, best practices, and support for our members" via the DSAIA website.

Director Deanna Tharpe says, "The local Down syndrome organization is one of the most important long-term support resources for families. But more than that, a local group also serves the educators, the medical professionals, extended family, and the community. A well-run DSA is about ongoing lifetime support and resources, friendly faces, and opportunities to gather, learn, and share with others. DSAIA then connects group leaders to others who can share experiences and information.

"And, I have to tell you, it's kind of amazing. Of course, we're also friendly faces who are happy to listen and offer support. However, the support comes in the form of training in the areas of nonprofit governance and operations. It comes in the form of information about effective programs, new technology and tools, and ways to save or raise funds."

OUR EXPERIENCE: Connections

[Our local DSA] helped connect us to other families. They offer classes for early childhood education information, potty training, starting school, finances, and so much more! They have an adult program (life skills and teaching independence), a club 21 group (parties and events for adult members), new member baskets, [and] summer pool and Christmas parties! They are a great advocate for inclusion in our community and they love Speed, our son, as much as we do!

—STEVIE RODRIGUEZ

A Need in Your Area?

Don't forget one last option: You! Every group started somewhere with someone. If there is a need in your area, it may be up to you to gather parents and get a group going. The DSAIA can help you with solutions on how to get started.

National and International Advocacy Organizations

There are many national/international registered non-profit groups that advocate for people with Down syndrome and their families. These groups often work together on large issues, legislation, and research funding. For example, a recent cooperative legislative accomplishment for these national organizations was the passing of the ABLE Act.

Why the ABLE Act?

Joe Meares, the founder and former chairperson of DADS, pointed out in a course on advocacy, "As a society, we determined years ago that certain people deserve a 'safety net,' then we forced them into poverty." The ABLE Act aims to change this. According to the NDSS website, "The ABLE Act would amend Section 529 of the Internal Revenue Service Code of 1986 to create tax-free savings accounts for individuals with disabilities." Basically the bill allows people with Down syndrome and other qualifying disabilities to open a tax-free savings account to prepare for expenses like college or other education, housing, and transportation, without jeopardizing their current or future eligibility for assistance with health care or supplemental income. There are, of course, caps on the eligibility and certain requirements about documentation and spending, however, over all it is a step toward helping people with disabilities plan for a more independent future.

The legislation was introduced in 2008 and required diligent advocacy and cooperation among several disability groups to bring it to the signing date by President Obama in December 2014. The next step is that each state must pass the legislation. Virginia was the first state to pass ABLE in March 2015. To find out the status of passing this legislation and opening an ABLE account in your state, contact the NDSS Director of State Government Affairs or your local Down syndrome organization.

Next Up on the Hill

Here are two of the many legislative issues that are currently being pursued by national and local advocates:

1. **Keeping All Students Safe in Schools Act (H.R. 1893).** This legislation prevents any school that receives federal funds to engage in using the disciplinary actions of restraint or seclusion in the school environment. Any action that threatens the student's safety or health will be deemed illegal and could result in funding consequences for the school and its district. You may be surprised to know that seclusion and restraint of children in the schools isn't technically illegal already and there are schools across the country with questionable discipline/teaching practices regarding children with disabilities. This is why, for your own child's safety, consider including a "No Restraint Letter" as a matter of course in your child's IEP.
2. The Trisomy 21 Research Resource Act of 2011 and the Trisomy 21 Research Centers of Excellence Act of 2011. Introduced by Rep. Cathy McMorris Rodgers (R-WA), co-

chair of the Congressional Down Syndrome Caucus, these two pieces of legislation aim to take Down syndrome research to the next level. Despite the prevalence of Down syndrome, research for treatments has lagged behind that for other medical conditions. "These bills would ensure that Down syndrome research remains on par with the research infrastructure of other diseases," says Rep. McMorris Rodgers. (Research is also a large component to advocacy and is discussed further in the next section of this chapter.) Although these were introduced in 2011, they remain a legislative priority for our national advocates.

There remain several other issues to be addressed on the local and national stages. For updates and action plans, sign up for NDSS advocacy alerts at *www.ndss.org/Advocacy/Advocacy-101/Advocacy-Alerts* and/or follow the NDSC Governmental Affairs page on Facebook: *www.facebook.com/dsadvocates*.

MY STORY: DAVID EGAN

No voice is more important than that of the self-advocate. In 2015, the Joseph P. Kennedy Jr. Foundation Public Policy Fellowship, a grant giving the recipient exposure to the process of federal policy-making, was awarded to David Egan. Mr. Egan is a longtime self-advocate on local and national affairs and is the first person with a developmental disability to be awarded this honor and responsibility. In the short video entitled "The Advocate, David Egan," Mr. Egan said, "I think we have to impact the world in some way; we want to leave a mark in this world. We want to make sure the world knows why we matter." He goes on to say, "That's where I want to be remembered, as someone who was a constant reminder that something great is happening. I'm just living my life as an example to transform other people's lives." (Watch the full video at http://moments.org/watch/david-egan.*)*

***

Legislative changes require local and national groups to work together and rally all of the community. There are also other awareness, educational, and support areas in which each Ds group has unique strengths to offer to families and self-advocates. The following list is alphabetical and includes the organization's name, mission, its main website page, and a couple of notes to give you a brief idea of how each organization works to improve the lives of those involved in the Down syndrome community. Disclaimer: this list does not equal endorsement, and conversely, if an organization is not on this list, it may be just as worthwhile, certainly worth investigating, and have potential for your support.

The Arc:

"The Arc promotes and protects the human rights of people with intellectual and developmental disabilities and actively supports their full inclusion and participation in the community throughout their lifetimes." Find online at *www.thearc.org*.

- "Being a part of The Arc means connecting with a broad community of people that have built this movement, fighting for inclusion in the classroom, workplace, and community; advocating for landmark laws like the Americans with Disabilities Act; and supporting each other through the triumphs and setbacks that occur in all families, including those with a member who has a disability. The Arc is a valuable resource for new parents learning the ropes, and it's these new families that will shape the future of The Arc and the disability movement as a whole for the next sixty-five years and beyond." —Peter Berns, CEO of The Arc

- National Center on Criminal Justice and Disability: *www.thearc.org/NCCJD* is a national clearinghouse for information and training on the topic of people with I/DD as victims, witnesses, and suspects or offenders of crime, developed and implemented in cooperation with legal professionals, by The Arc of the U.S.

Dads Appreciating Down Syndrome (DADS)

Dads Appreciating Down Syndrome is "a committee or community group (within a local Down syndrome support organization) of fathers of children who happen to have Down syndrome. We hesitate to call [ourselves] a 'support group,' even though we do, in many ways, support each other." Find online at *http://dadsnational.org*.

- Members come together in monthly meetings for discussion and contact.
- The group prides itself in being able to answer questions. "Ask A D.A.D. is a quick-response forum designed to get fathers' questions answered quickly (within 24 hours)." See *http://dadsnational.org/ask-a-dad.html*.

Down Syndrome Diagnosis Network (DSDN)

The group's mission: "The Down Syndrome Diagnosis Network (DSDN) supports families with current information and real-life accounts of life with Down syndrome during the prenatal to early childhood phases. DSDN is committed to facilitating unbiased, family-centered discussion of Down syndrome within the medical community. We strive to cultivate a culture of acceptance and inclusion for people with Down syndrome at all stages of life." Find online at *www.dsdiagnosisnetwork.org*.

The group's president, Heather Bradley, says, "Our primary goal at DSDN is to provide up-to-date information and support to families following a diagnosis. We especially look to serve those that do not have a local organization or are not ready to get involved locally yet."

- DSDN provides small, private online groups in birth-club style from pregnancy and aids families in getting connected locally with organizations and families.
- The group assists parents in providing feedback to physicians about how the diagnosis was delivered.

Down Syndrome Education (DSE)

Their mission: "Our goal is to improve outcomes for all children with Down syndrome, helping them to lead more independent, productive, and fulfilling lives." Find online at *www.dseusa.org/en-us*.

- The group has conducted controlled trials of targeted interventions for children with Down syndrome. They found that carefully structured daily reading and language teaching can improve reading and language development for primary-school children with Down syndrome. They are publishing a handbook to help with this, one that can be used in schools around the world.
- Check the events page for ongoing education events to help parents and educators: *www.dseusa.org/en-us/events*.

Down Syndrome International (DSi)

Down Syndrome International is based in the UK. Its mission: "to improve quality of life for people with Down syndrome worldwide and promote their inherent right to be accepted and included as valued and equal members of their communities." Find online at *www.ds-int.org*.

- The group hosts the World Down Syndrome Congress every three years: *www.ds-int.org/world-down-syndrome-congress*.
- DSi coordinates the WDSD website (as a single global meeting place to share WDSD world events); the WDSD global video event "Let Us In!"; the WDSD conference held at the United Nations Headquarters in New York, USA, on 21 March; the "Lots of Socks" campaign; and the WDSD Awards.

Down Syndrome Medical Interest Group (DSMIG-USA)

DSMIG-USA is a group of health professionals committed to promoting the optimal health care and wellness of individuals with Ds across the lifespan. Find online at *http://dsmig-usa.org*.

- Members of DSMIG-USA are professionals from a variety of disciplines who provide care to individuals with Down syndrome and/or their families.
- To accomplish its mission, DSMIG endeavors to educate professionals on the latest research and comprehensive care regarding Ds. It facilitates networking among health professionals caring for individuals with Ds, supports development of Ds clinics, and works to identify and disseminate best practices of care.

Global Down Syndrome Foundation (GDSF)

The mission: "Our goal is to significantly improve the lives of people with Down syndrome through research, medical care, education, and advocacy. We work to educate governments, educational organizations, and society in order to affect legislative and social changes so that every person with Down syndrome has an equitable chance at a satisfying life." Find online at *www.globaldownsyndrome.org*.

- GDSF has brought attention to the fact that Down syndrome is the least funded genetic condition by the National Institutes of Health (NIH) and has taken steps to continue to spotlight the need for research, raise funds, enable grants, and push for a better quality of life for people with Down syndrome throughout their lifespan.
- GDSF opened the Sie Center in Colorado to patients with Down syndrome in November of 2010. It is located at Children's Hospital Colorado, where there is a spectrum of experts to draw from. Most importantly, the Sie Center is comprised of a multidisciplinary "Dream Team" of experts with more than eighty years of combined experience in caring for children with Down syndrome and developmental disabilities.

International Down Syndrome Coalition (IDSC)

The International Down Syndrome Coalition is "dedicated to helping and advocating for individuals with Down syndrome from conception and throughout life. We promote the dignity and respect of individuals with Ds and assist the families who love them. We provide support, education, and connection to other families as well as to local resources. The IDSC operates and advocates independent of any political cause or religious affiliation and we welcome all to our community." Find online at *http://theidsc.org*.

"The IDSC connects families to each other and to local resources. Our Facebook groups serve more than 15,000 families. We have groups by age, diagnosis and other demographic profiles. We connect those families to each other and we introduce them to local resources - their local Down syndrome organizations, local Arc, etc. We also host a meet up at 13 locations across the United States and Canada where more than 500 families spend the weekend together."
—Beth Sullivan, IDSC Chairperson

- The IDSC facilitates parent conversations in private group forums via Facebook areas specific to the family's situation. Find the listing here: *http://theidsc.org/resources*.
- The IDSC offers adoption grants to families domestically adopting children with Down syndrome.

International Mosaic Down Syndrome Association (IMDSA)

The International Mosaic Down Syndrome Association is "designed to support any family or individual whose life has been touched by mosaic Down syndrome by continuously pursuing research opportunities and increasing awareness in the medical, educational, and public communities throughout the world." Find online at *www.imdsa.org*.

- The group holds a research and retreat weekend, including a youth camp: *www.imdsa.org/2015R&Rweekend*.
- The IMDSA maintains a toll-free hotline to help connect families to information and support. See *www.imdsa.org/aboutus*.

National Association for Down Syndrome (NADS)

The National Association for Down Syndrome "supports all persons with Down syndrome in achieving their full potential." Find online at *www.nads.org*.

- NADS sponsors a conference in Chicago every other year.
- Founded in 1960, NADS is the oldest organization in the United States serving children and adults with Down syndrome.

National Down Syndrome Adoption Network (NDSAN)

The National Down Syndrome Adoption Network says: "Our mission is to ensure that every child born with Down syndrome has the opportunity to grow up in a loving family." Find online at *www.ndsan.org*.

- The NDSAN is a nonprofit program that offers support and information to parents whose child has received a diagnosis of Down syndrome and may be considering an adoption plan for their child.
- The NDSAN would love to have more families like yours on their registry, who are interested in adopting a child with Down syndrome.

National Down Syndrome Congress (NDSC)

The National Down Syndrome Congress's mission: "The purpose of the NDSC is to promote the interests of people with Down syndrome and their families through advocacy, public awareness, and information. When we empower individuals and families from all demographic backgrounds, we reshape the way people understand and experience Down syndrome." Find online at *www.ndsccenter.org*.

"While we are best known as the 'convention people,' we really are much more than that. When parents contact us, we pride ourselves on spending time with them, providing them with individualized information, figuring out how best to help them with their unique circumstances, and referring them to resources closest to them."

—David Tolleson, NDSC Executive Director

- Each year, thousands of people from across the globe attend the National Down Syndrome Congress annual convention. See *www.ndsccenter.org/the-convention*.
- The group provides individualized support and information for new and expectant parents. You can call them at 1-800-232-6372 or e-mail (info@ndsccenter.org) for resources to best help you and your family!

National Down Syndrome Society (NDSS)

The National Down Syndrome Society says of its mission: "The mission of the National Down Syndrome Society is to be the national advocate for the value, acceptance, and inclusion of people with Down syndrome." Find online at *www.ndss.org*.

- The NDSS National Policy Center supports the mission of NDSS by advocating for federal, state, and local policies that positively impact people with Down syndrome across the country.
- The National Buddy Walk Program has grown from seventeen walks in 1995 to more than 250 this year! See *www.ndss.org/Buddy-Walk/About-the-National-Buddy-Walk-Program*.

The Special Olympics

The organization says, "The mission of Special Olympics is to provide year-round sports training and athletic competition in a variety of Olympic-type sports for children and adults with intellectual disabilities, giving them continuing opportunities to develop physical fitness, demonstrate courage, experience joy, and participate in a sharing of gifts, skills, and friendship with their families, other Special Olympics athletes, and the community." Find online at *www.specialolympics.org*.

- Special Olympics has become the largest global public health organization dedicated to serving people with intellectual disabilities.
- The organization provides coaching guides in many languages for the benefit of its athletes and their trainers.

OUR EXPERIENCE: Getting Involved

I am in no way politically savvy or well-connected. Never in a million years did I think I would ever care to be "in the know" of government politics. I grew up in a small town, with a close family. We felt invincible and seemingly un-phased by all that DC drama. Wouldn't touch it with a ten-foot pole. Wanted nothing to do with it. Never thought it would directly affect *my* life. Well, that changed pretty quickly the moment I first held Macy in my arms, looked deeply into her eyes, and fell immediately and unconditionally in love with this precious person.

I am now very aware that if you want change . . . you must get in the game. No longer can we sit on the sidelines and watch as decisions are being made that drastically impact the dreams of my daughter who deserves the right, just like everyone else, to live the American Dream. She, just like the next person, deserves to be treated with dignity and respect. I am thankful that organizations like [the] National Down Syndrome Society exist to help our daughter, and so many others just like her, to develop to their fullest potential, to ensure they become valued members of our community, and have the ability to lead truly fulfilling lives.

Now I am glad every time someone reaches out to me with questions regarding various legislative issues. I certainly do not pretend to have all the answers—after all, who does?! I tell people all the time, many of whom are initially intimidated and afraid to pick up that phone or shoot that e-mail to a lawmaker, that you do not have to [be] politically connected to help effect change in society; you simply have to be passionate and persistent!

– SHERRI HARNISCH, BOARD PRESIDENT, DOWN SYNDROME ALLIANCE OF THE MIDLANDS

Research

Modern advocacy and support requires more than awareness language. Solid research enables better health care, and confirms which educational and therapeutic methods and tools work best. Additionally, studies of both scientific and societal natures impact the direction of our national Down syndrome organizations and government institutions, showing what issues require focused attention and where there has been the greatest progress.

One substantial challenge facing research and potential research regarding Ds is the lack of funding. The Global Down Syndrome Foundation, in particular, references the funding disparities for research from the NIH and works to both rally for change from the government regarding attention and support and does extensive fundraising specifically toward the purpose of providing research grants for projects that will positively affect the lives of people with Down syndrome.

Note that none of the national groups are looking for "a cure for Down syndrome." Down syndrome is a human condition that occurs naturally at conception. "Down syndrome is a treatable disorder," said Dr. Edward McCabe, a renowned pediatrician and geneticist, before the UN on March 21st, 2012. "Most people born with trisomy 21 have physical ailments that are treatable and are treated successfully." In fact, the GDSF website specifies: "While the overwhelming majority of individuals with Down syndrome and their family members would want to improve the health outcomes of individuals with Down syndrome, including cognition, many families are offended by the word "cure" because the word is imbued with negative connotations." What researchers are aiming to achieve are better living conditions for a person with Down syndrome throughout his or her life. Research is critical to creating the medical improvements and treatment for physical conditions associated with Down syndrome.

Research studies are also important to addressing and creating societal and educational improvements, for example, studies on the impact of full integration of people with Ds in schools and community have been an influential factor in increasing access for students with Down syndrome. Research is both a form of advocacy on its own, and also enables advocacy within the previously mentioned forums of medical, educational, and policy-making communities. Most of the national organizations support, either monetarily or through advocacy, research projects that help those living with Down syndrome, but there are a few organizations that include research as a key priority to their mission.

Linda Crnic Institute for Down Syndrome

The Linda Crnic Institute for Down Syndrome is an affiliate of the GDSF and the first academic home for Down syndrome research in the United States. The mission of the Crnic Institute is to significantly improve the lives of people with Down syndrome by eradicating the medical and cognitive ill effects associated with the condition. See *www.ucdenver.edu/academics/colleges/medicalschool/institutes/lindacrnic/Pages*.

LuMind Foundation

The mission of the LuMind Foundation is to stimulate biomedical research that will accelerate the development of treatments to significantly improve cognition, including memory, learning, and speech, for individuals with Down syndrome so they: participate more successfully in school, lead more active and independent lives, and avoid the early onset of Alzheimer's disease. Find online at *www.lumindfoundation.org*.

DS-Connect

DS-Connect is a voluntary, confidential, online survey that collects basic health information about people with Down syndrome, and is one result of the National Institutes of Health (NIH) Down Syndrome Consortium, which is a working group founded in 2006 that includes scientists from across the NIH, advocates from national Down syndrome groups, self-advocates, and medical professionals.

Down Syndrome Consortium

According to the NIH website, "The Working Group was charged with coordinating ongoing research already supported by the NIH related to Down syndrome, and to enhance new, NIH-supported research efforts. The Working Group, with input from the outside scientific and family communities and at the request of Congress, created the NIH Research Plan on Down Syndrome in 2007 to focus on genetic and neurobiological research relating to the cognitive dysfunction and the progressive late-life dementia associated with the condition. The plan aimed to build upon ongoing NIH-supported research on Down syndrome, reflect the changing lives of the individuals and families affected, and take advantage of emerging scientific opportunities. After several years of working with scientific and family communities to achieve the various goals of the plan, the NIH created the Down Syndrome Consortium to foster communication and idea-sharing among the NIH, individuals with Down syndrome and their families, national organizations interested in Down syndrome, and pediatric and other organizations."

A simple way to help or even be a part of current research for bettering the quality of life for people with Down syndrome is to include your loved one with Down syndrome in the Down syndrome registry. Just by being a part of the registry and updating health information annually allows for researchers to see as a conglomerate the health conditions of people with Down syndrome so that they can identify trends and areas of need that will benefit the Ds community and consequently analyze the positive (or negative) effects of new treatments or medications. This is the only national registry of people with Down syndrome, and it is completely voluntary. Even within the registry there are levels of information that you can choose to give and/or receive.

Why Connect?

George Capone, MD, director of the Down Syndrome Clinic at the Kennedy Krieger Institute, says, "Ds-Connect allows people to participate from all corners of the globe. They all answer the same kinds of health questions and that permits researchers to identify similarities, differences, and important trends in the population that may then be the basis for further, more focused, research studies." (Watch full video here at: *https://dsconnect.nih.gov*.)

There are also personal benefits to joining the registry. For parents, it offers a secure online space for health history and information, printable as a summary for your records or for doctors' reference (there is even an option to upload attachments of more detailed reports or information to keep on file). It enables you to access a family-driven list of health-care providers in your area. Input and follow your child's growth measurements and compare to others with Down syndrome. Plus, if you choose to, you can learn about current and new research studies for improving the quality of life for people with Down syndrome. Connect with scientists who study Down syndrome. Help scientists develop new or more effective treatments for people with Down syndrome.

Recent Progress from New Research

There are many exciting developments in the current research into Ds. Researchers who are technically outside of the "Down syndrome community" are starting to take note of the anomalies with trisomy 21 that could lead to answers that will help the larger, typical, population fight these and other medical challenges. For example, some researchers believe the key to curing both Alzheimer's disease and childhood leukemia may be discovered through research connected to trisomy 21. There continue to be positive secrets to unlock that can benefit all of humanity that appear to be connected to the twenty-first chromosome.

Chapter Eleven
A Worldwide Network of Friends

Have you ever noticed that when you're thinking about buying a new car, you start seeing cars you'd like to have everywhere? Or once you got pregnant, there were babies everywhere? Your eyes have now opened up to the beautiful people with Down syndrome. This chapter will point out how people with Down syndrome are becoming included in the arts and media. We'll also introduce you to a few of the countless connections available on the Internet, including the chance to add your own voice.

The Media and Arts

Art imitates life. People with Down syndrome are now included in the classroom, in the workforce, and in the community at large. No longer hidden from their neighbors, they also shine for the camera.

Television and Movies

Perhaps you've seen some of the people with Down syndrome featured on popular television shows, such as Lauren Potter on *Glee* and Jamie Brewer on *American Horror Story*. Then there's the big screen with new stars like David DeSanctis in the 2015 feature film *Where Hope Grows*. Two self-advocates, Sam and Mattie, are working as writers and producers of *A Zombie Movie*. They raised over $68,000 for the project via Kickstarter, and production has begun.

Other actors like Connor Long are also moving up the ranks with independent films and stage productions. Long has several movies in the can and more on the way. After a screening of the short film *Menschen*, there was a Q & A segment with the audience, and self-advocate and actress in local theater Jenny Koley stated she was glad to see Connor Long in the movie. She said, "Connor has Down syndrome, like me. I don't hide it. I'm proud of it." This is a sentiment that the movie's director, Sarah Lotfi, has heard in other screenings across the country. Connor's currently involved in a live-action short entitled *Learning to Drive*, planned for release in early 2016.

Abilities, Not Disabilities

In the 2015 WDSD video created and shared on The Mighty, DeSanctis said, "If I can remember 130 lines for my part in the movie, then can't you see my abilities? Not my disabilities?"

Music

Around the world people with Down syndrome are making noise. In the case of the Finnish punk band, PKN (Pertti Kurikan Nimipäivät), they made a lot of noise this year at Eurovision 2015. (At the time of this writing they are semi-finalists—an amazing accomplishment for anyone.)

Books

Of course, there are also authors with Down syndrome as well: *Count Us In*, for instance, by Jason Kingsley and Mitchell Levitz, written about their life, friendship, and experiences. *The North Side of Down* is a co-memoir written by Amanda Bailey and her sister Nancy Bailey, covering trauma and triumph. Not every writer with Ds writes about Down syndrome, for example my son, Marcus Sikora, released his first story-book and animated short for children, *Black Day: The Monster Rock Band* in the summer of 2015. He indicated in an interview published on The Huffington Post that Down syndrome, "Doesn't have anything to do with the book."

Advertising

Then there are the advertising models. Maybe you've seen Izzy in the Target ad. In Canada, a toddler named Pip made a splash with an amazing billboard. "What makes you different is what makes you beautiful." Pip's mom said she pursued this because she wants to help everyone to see: "People first, disability second."

2015 New York Fashion Week Diversifies

Actress Jamie Brewer is noted for her work on the series *American Horror Story*. In 2015, she also took to the catwalk as the first person with Down syndrome to be included as a model in the New York Fashion Week. Brewer wore a gown designed by Carrie Hammer and used this opportunity to share with the media that anything is possible.

Changing the Face of Beauty is just one of the many voices calling for people of varied abilities to be included in advertising campaigns. In 2015 they began the #ImReady campaign with the goal of getting fifteen new advertisers to include people with Ds or other disabilities in their advertising. As of May 2015 there are more than 100 companies who have answered this challenge and have committed to inclusion of people with Down syndrome or other disabilities in their advertising and media. "The thought of working with 100 companies passionate about seeing all their customers was a dream and it is now a reality," says the campaign founder, Katie Driscoll.

The consequence of media integration of people with Down syndrome in TV, movies, and advertising speaks to the overall increasing of acceptance of more diverse communities as well as filling the need for visible positive role models for people with Down syndrome to dream big and pursue.

MY STORY: CONNOR LONG

Connor is a twenty-year-old award-winning actor, honored for his role in the live-action short film Menschen. *Not yet rich and famous, but he's trying. Check out his video promoting his next project:* www.youtube.com/watch?v=W77Xr7Kn_kw.

He's also a headline-garnering advocate. The Denver Post *reported, "Connor Long honored for commitment to helping those with Down syndrome." Connor said "Thank you" in three languages as part of his acceptance speech at the GDSF ceremony.*

In his spare time, between his two jobs at a local cantina and boutique, auditioning for and acting in films, he is going to ride in the Courage Classic, a thirty-three-mile bike ride in the Colorado mountains. I could have filled in much of Connor's story from his online publicity and interviews. Fortunately for me (and you), Connor gave me some time on FaceTime to chat about what's going on for him now and next.

On what he likes to do with friends: "I like hanging out. Watching films. Singing with them. Bowling, of course." To which he added, "I bowl perfectly."

On what's coming up: "There's still work to do on a current film project, Learning to Drive. *The state Special Olympics meet for swimming and the Courage Classic."*

On his part time jobs (a boutique and a cantina): "I bus tables; I clean dishes." Also, "I do like it. It's my favorite restaurant."

On asking about friends at work, well, here he broke into song. (I wish I had a video of this interview.)

On what's next: "Keep acting. [I] want to be in a 'Power Ranger' or in that kind of movie, action and entertainment." This is why he is also taking tae kwon do classes.

On advice to new parents: "Trust is the key to raising a baby with Down syndrome."

***

Blogs and Online Groups

In this day and age, when you join any new community, it can quickly become a worldwide group. This is not only a clear advantage to people in rural areas; online groups and resources are also a great help to those anxious about meeting others in person, who have work hours that are not conducive to support groups, who want information more than personal correspondence or interaction, and on. Also online support and information can help people whose circumstances feel very specific. We usually find there are others in the same boat as us, even if the "boat" is spread across states, counties, even countries.

Online Support Groups

Some organizations specialize in online support for new parents. For example:

- The DSDN connects people via small, private online groups in birth-club style from pregnancy through age three.
- The IDSC administrates and promotes specific private Facebook support groups for parents at every level of their children's life.
- BabyCenter.com has boards for online interaction and both prenatal and postnatal information for mothers and families who care for a child with Down syndrome.

Another subset of the Down syndrome community is adults with Down syndrome and their families. In 2013 Stephanie Holland created a website specifically to serve and facilitate conversations with families of adults with Down syndrome. The site is called The Road We've Shared.

OUR EXPERIENCE: Creating The Road We've Shared

I am a single mother who stays at home to care for my adult son (twenty-seven) who has Down syndrome. When the woman who helped me become an advocate lost her own son to a tragic, senseless death, I turned to social media in that time of grief. Ethan Saylor died in police custody over the price of a movie ticket (#JusticeForEthan). In the months that followed, a group of parents who did not know each other, from all over the world, came together in a real grassroots effort to support my friend and advocate for change.

We are scattered across the U.S., but our hearts couldn't be more in sync. It became clear to us that the existing Down syndrome organizations appealed more to parents of young children and focused on topics that were no longer relevant in our lives, so I decided to create my own community. Now, we are growing a safe place for open dialog which will not only provide support and friendship but also necessary information and resources for the families of adults with Ds.

I have an MA in disability studies so my passion is to create something useful while satisfying a personal desire to establish a social historical record of what life on "The Road" has been like for this generation of trailblazers.

—STEPHANIE HOLLAND

Variety of Missions and Voices

When we're talking about blogs and Facebook pages, the voices, faces, stories, and missions vary. There are informative blogs; for example, DownSyndromePrenatalTesting.com, by Mark Leach, is primarily information based on, you guessed it, prenatal testing. DisabilityScoop.com is an online newspaper: "the premier source for developmental disability news." David Perry blogs *How Did We Get Into This Mess?* at ThisMess.net and tackles issues of ableism, disability, and the "Cult of Compliance." OllieBean.com offers information and blogs across disabilities with items and opinions pertinent to our community.

There are more, many more, some with broader and some more specific information.

Families Blogging

Families often find that blogging is a great way to connect with others, share news and photos with their families, and advocate for their child. The advantages to reading family blogs are several. First is the diversity of stories. Every family and every child is unique, and reading blogs by various parents at various stages of a person's life, it's easy to see this fact. There are families who adopt children. There are families with several children. There are families with one child. There are prenatal diagnosis stories and postnatal diagnosis stories. There are families that grieve and families that celebrate. The medical issues range across the spectrum, as well as how those families cope with those medical issues. Most importantly, what everyone can learn is that people with Down syndrome are as diverse as the human condition.

One mom, Meriah Nichols, created DownSyndromeBlogs.org, and anyone can peruse the Down syndrome blog site categories ranging from schooling, to age of child, to religious categories.

Voices Equal Awareness

It's astonishing and enlightening to read these stories of people with Down syndrome. How they are loved. How they live in their communities, schools, work, and family. These stories themselves and the emotions they can generate are a very important component to awareness and advocacy. It's yet another way we all connect to the broader community. You may choose to add your story, as well. In fact, you can share from a blog or share just one story on the website ADayInTheLifeWithDownSyndrome.com. As well, there are bloggers connecting from all over the world, sharing a common voice to share the value of the lives of people with Down syndrome.

Made in the USA
Las Vegas, NV
15 November 2024